CAREGIVER & PROFESSIONAL GUIDE

Purpose of This Book

This story invites children to share what "home" feels like to them, especially if they've witnessed yelling, arguing, or other frightening behavior between adults.

It functions as a gentle, child-friendly risk assessment to help identify possible adverse childhood experiences and guide appropriate support.

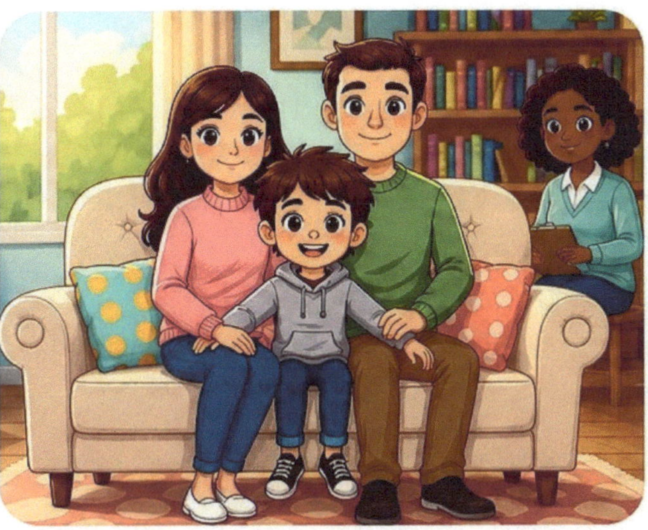

A child does not need to name what is happening at home to need support.
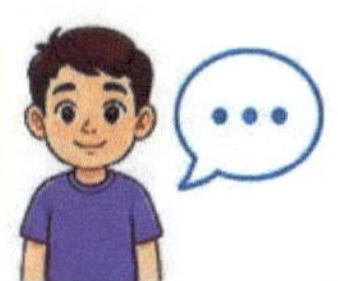

What This Book Helps You Notice

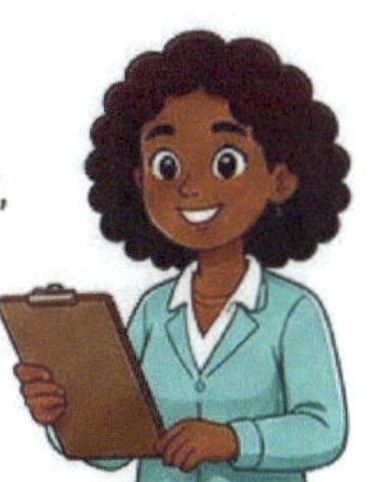

As you read with a child, pay close attention to how they respond, not just what they say.

This book is designed to help you gently notice signs of how a child may be feeling or coping.

You may notice:

Emotional responses

- Changes in mood such as sad, worried, quiet, or upset
- Hesitation, avoidance, or discomfort with certain pages
- Relief or increased engagement during safe or calming moments

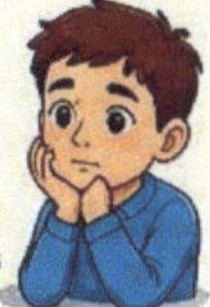

Body cues

- Tension in the body such as stiffness or fidgeting
- Covering eyes or ears
- Becoming still, withdrawn, or overly alert

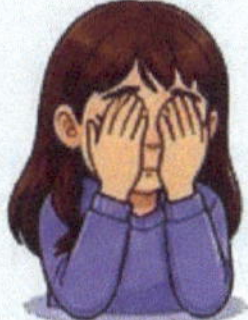

Behavioral cues

- Skipping pages or changing the subject
- Wanting to stay on certain pages longer
- Becoming clingy or seeking reassurance

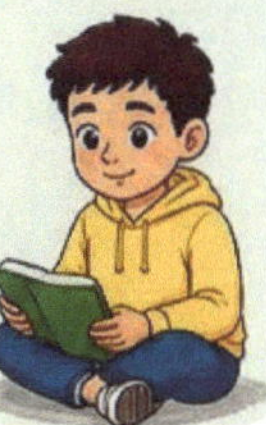

Verbal responses

- Sharing personal experiences or stories
- Using strong or emotional language
- Mentioning fear, conflict, or things happening at home

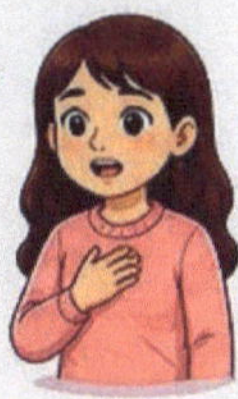

Important: These responses are not conclusions. They are gentle clues that may help guide supportive conversations.

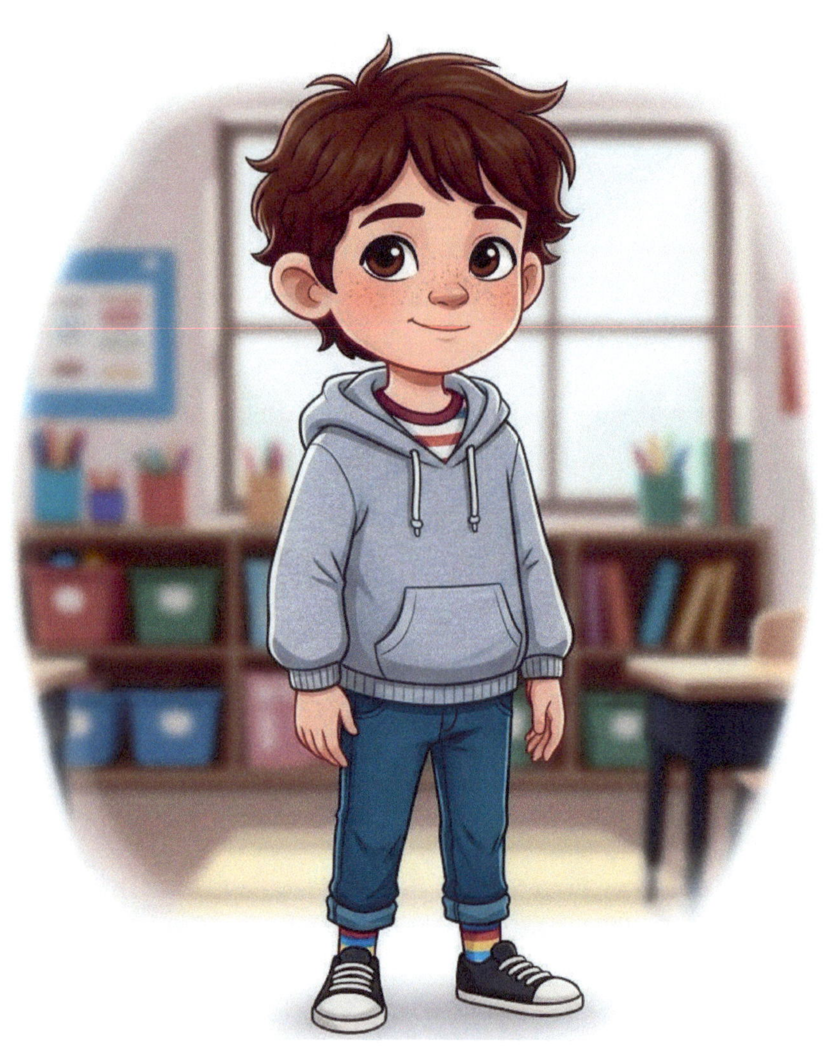

Hi! My name's Grayson, and I just started school. That means I'm a big kid now! School is super fun, but it can be a little scary too, especially when you don't have a lot of friends yet.

Do you have friends at school?

Today I sat in my favorite spot in class, right by the window. I love looking at the people walking outside and the dogs playing in the park. I even made a new friend on the playground!

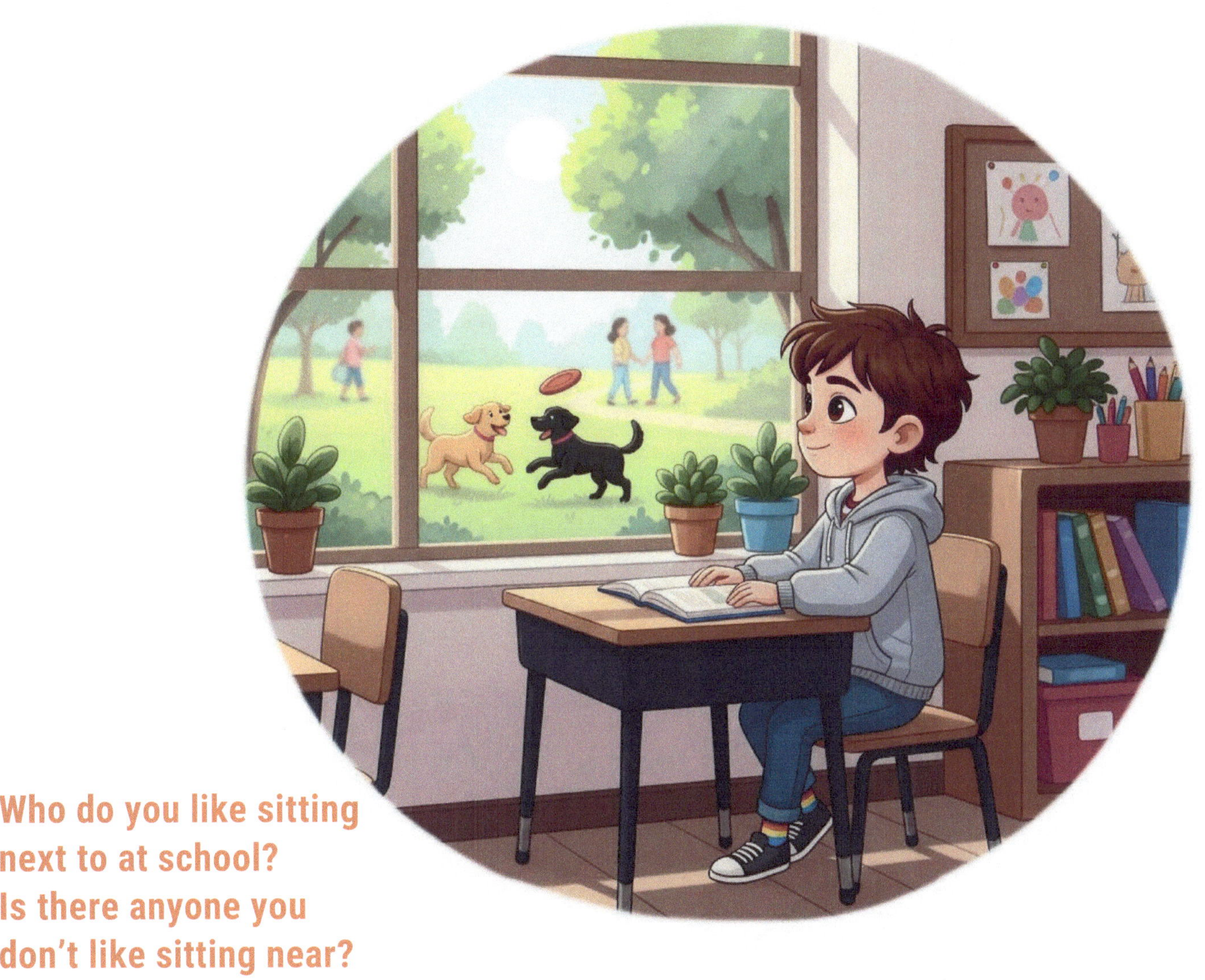

My new friend Alex likes the same games I do. His favorite is basketball, just like mine.

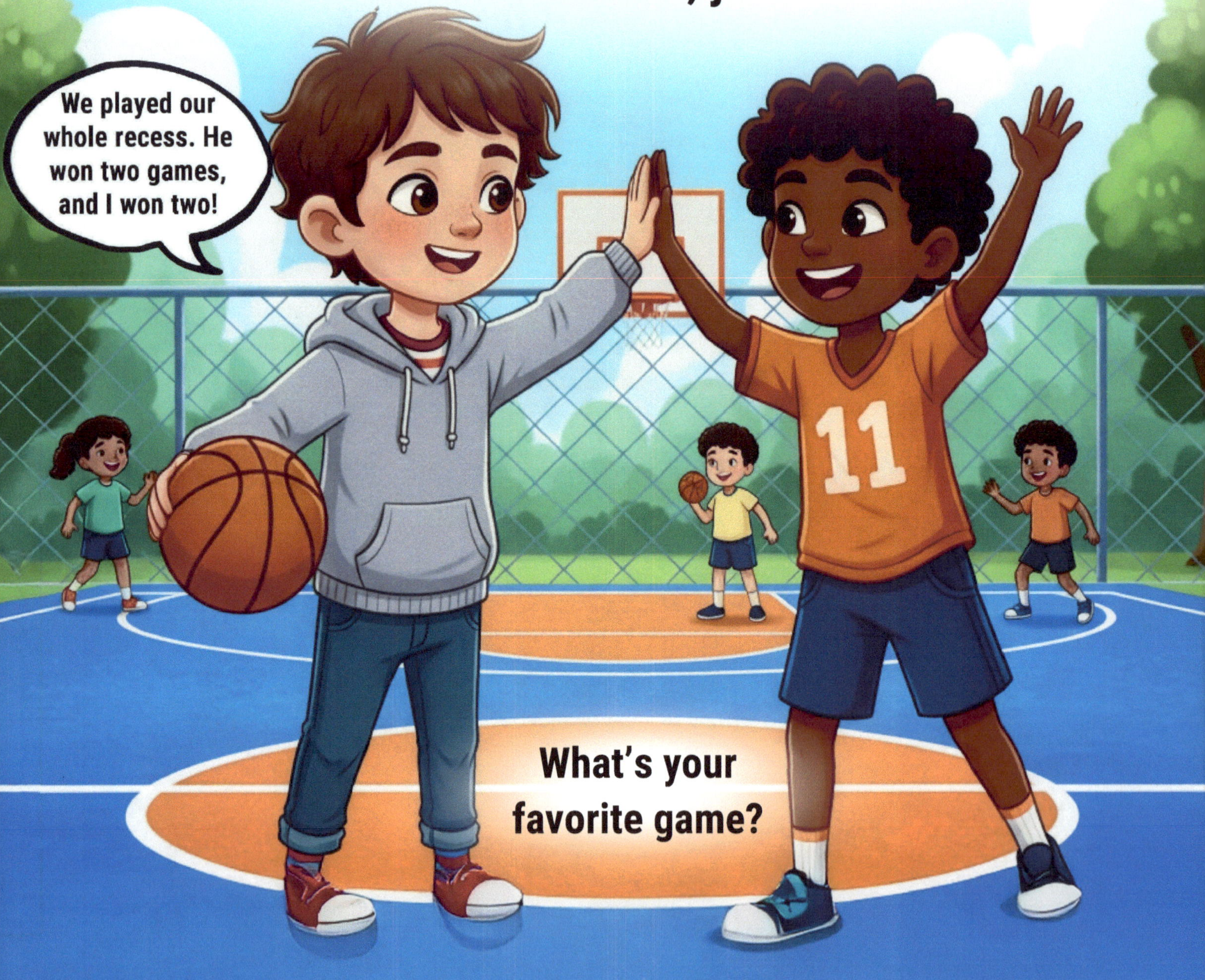

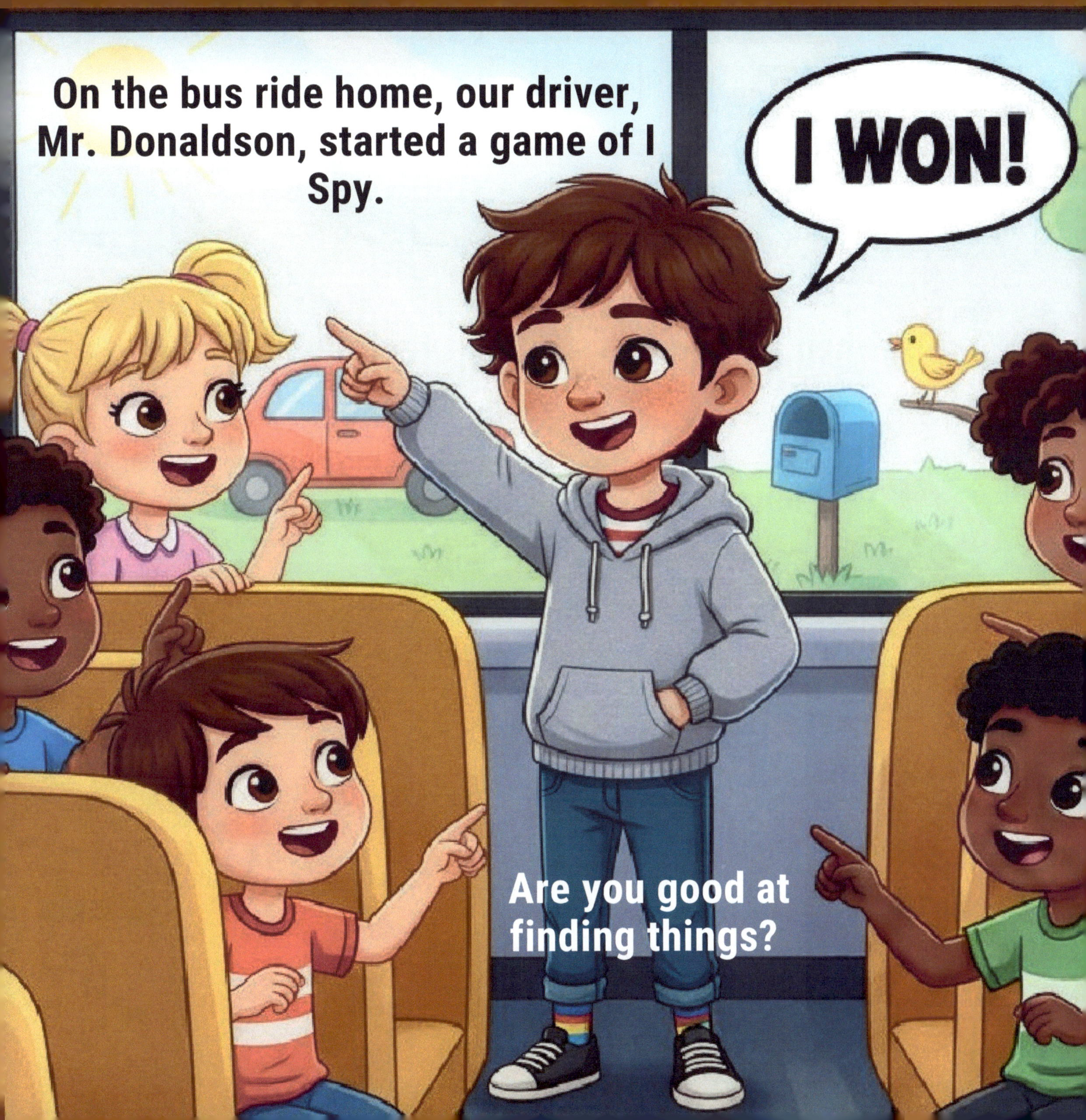

On the bus ride home, our driver, Mr. Donaldson, started a game of I Spy.
I WON!
Are you good at finding things?

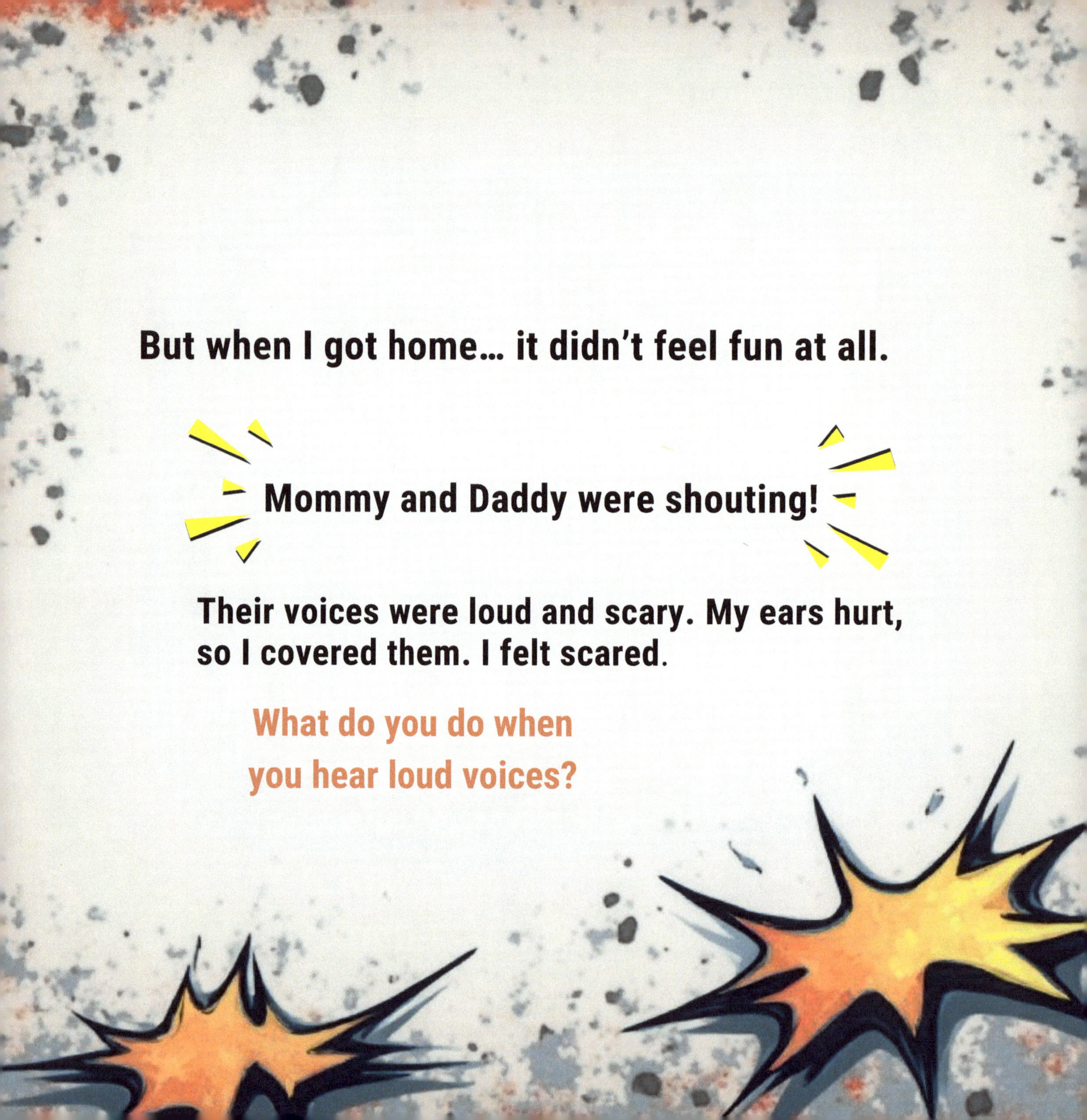

But when I got home... it didn't feel fun at all.

Mommy and Daddy were shouting!

Their voices were loud and scary. My ears hurt, so I covered them. I felt scared.

What do you do when you hear loud voices?

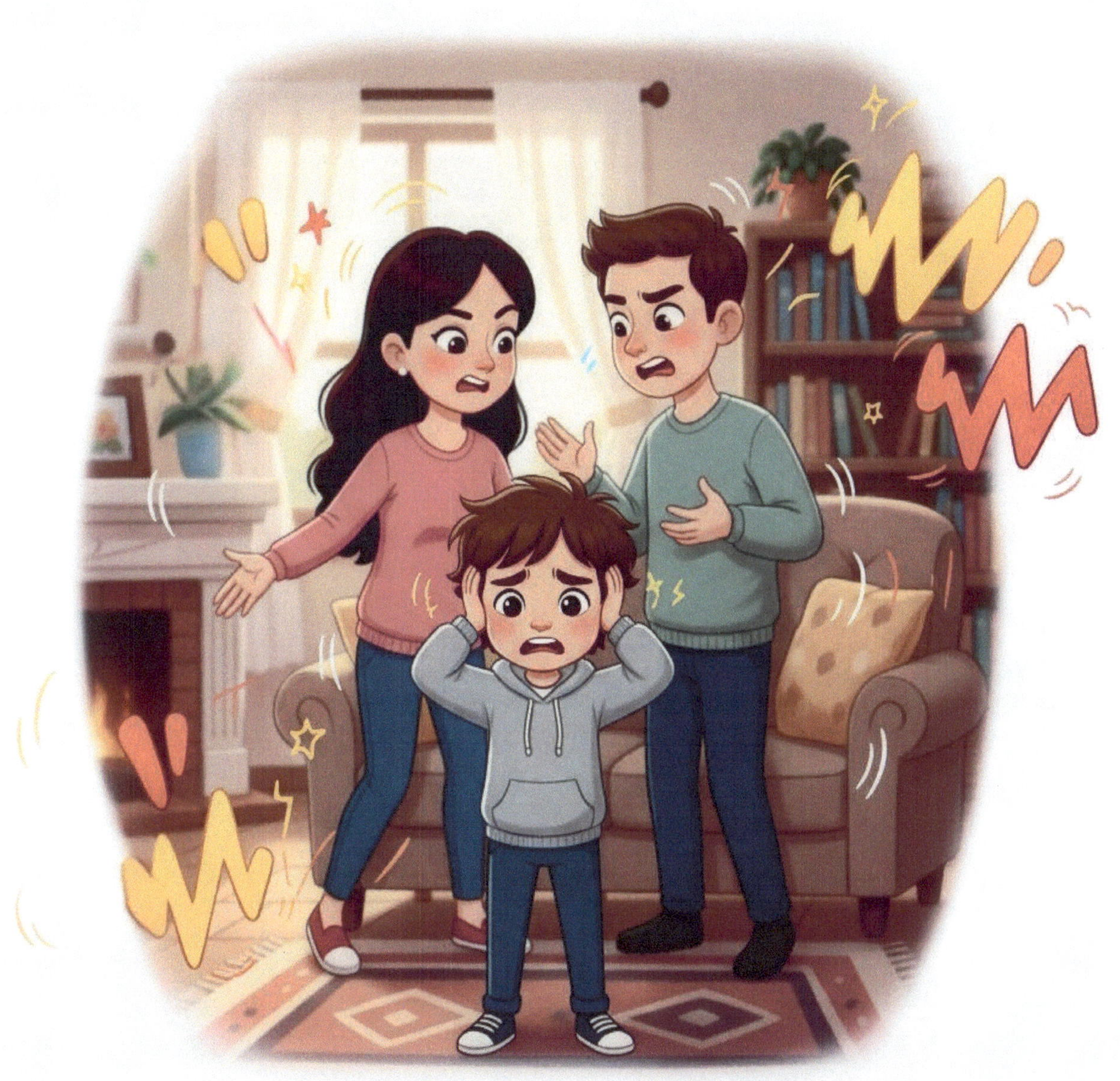

Have you ever heard loud or angry voices at home? How did it make you feel?

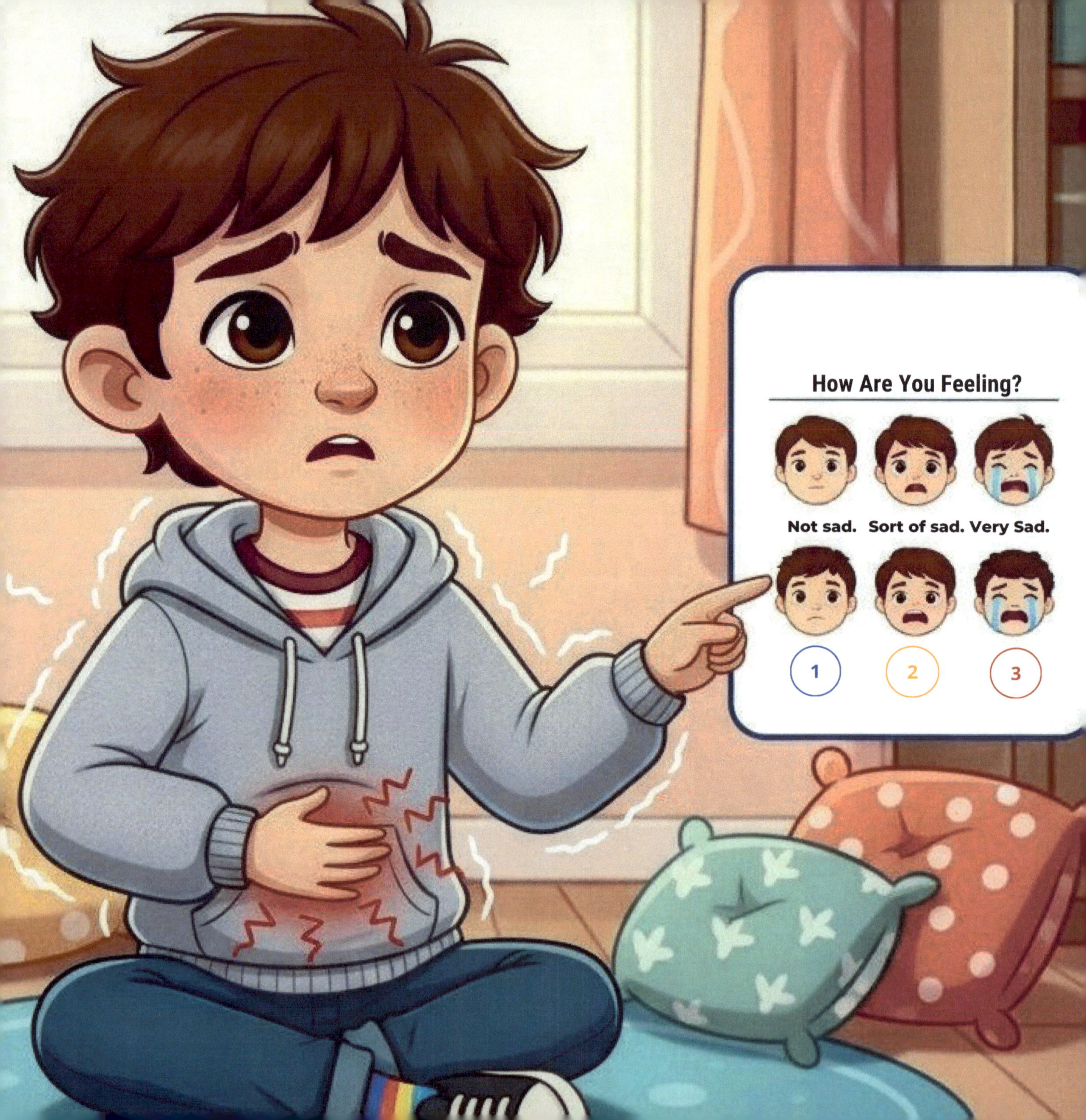
How Are You Feeling?
Not sad.
Sort of sad.
Very Sad.
1
2
3

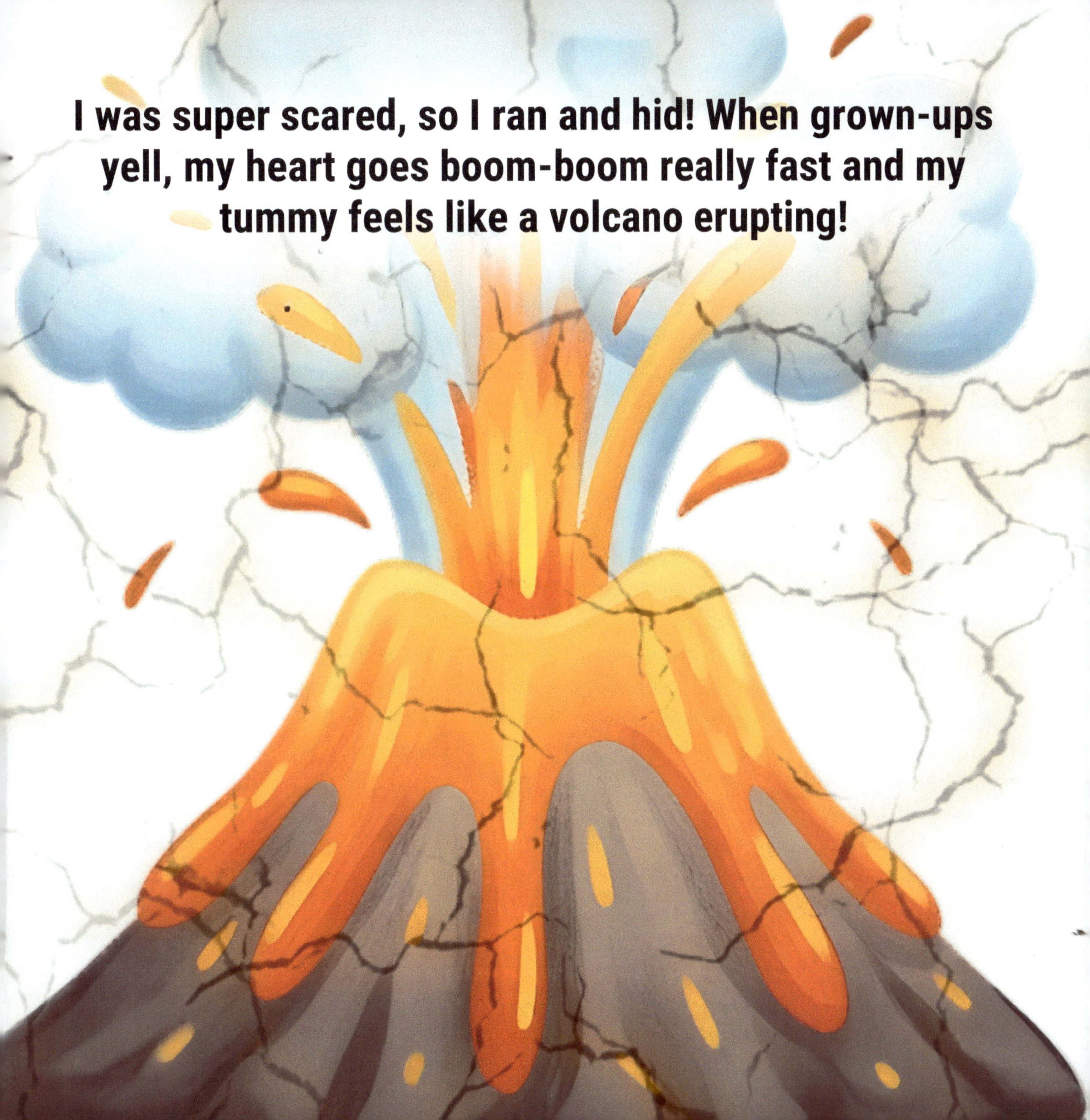
I was super scared, so I ran and hid! When grown-ups yell, my heart goes boom-boom really fast and my tummy feels like a volcano erupting!

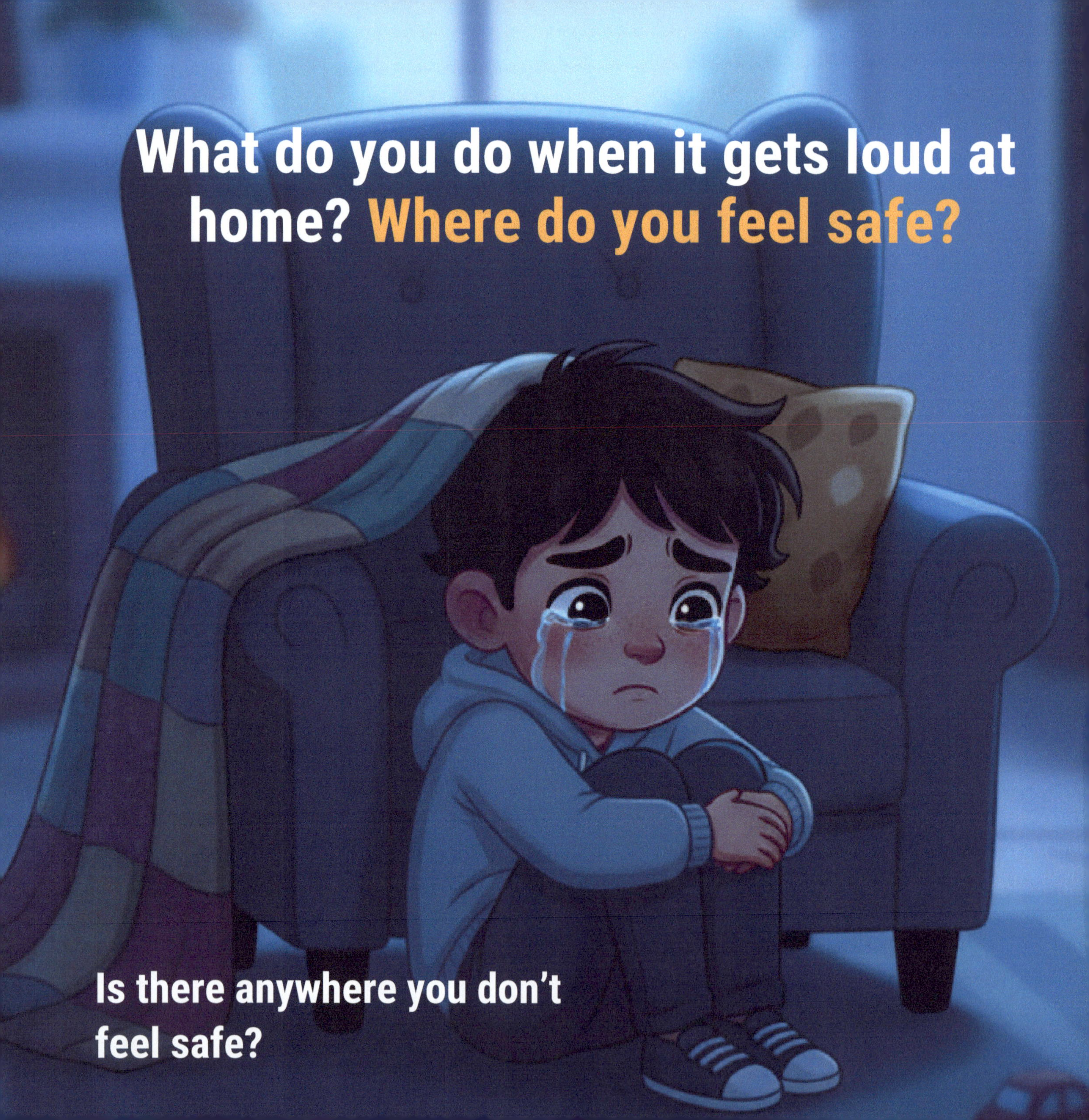

What do you do when it gets loud at home? Where do you feel safe?
Is there anywhere you don't feel safe?

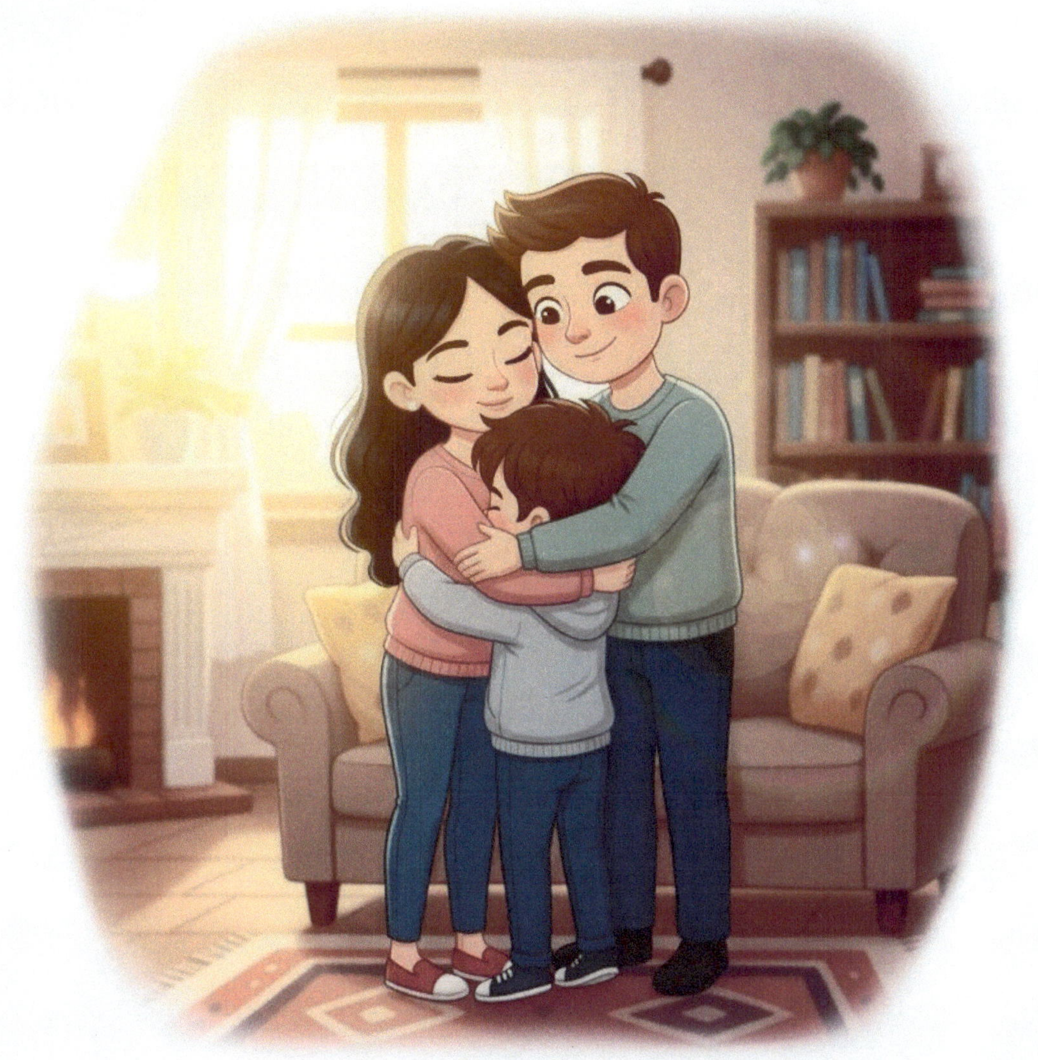

I feel safe when Mommy and Daddy use gentle voices.

What makes you feel safe?

Sometimes, after I hear yelling at home, I have scary dreams about monsters who shout and stomp.

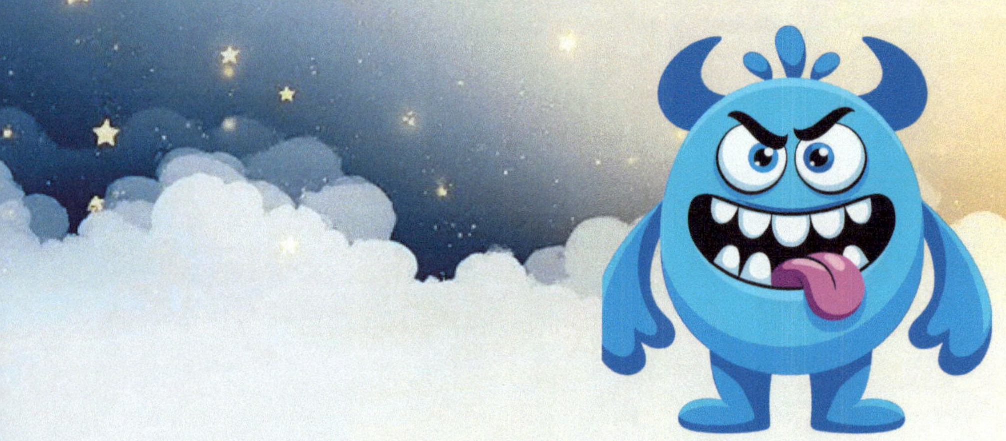

In my dreams, I try to open my eyes, but it's hard. Do you ever have scary dreams?

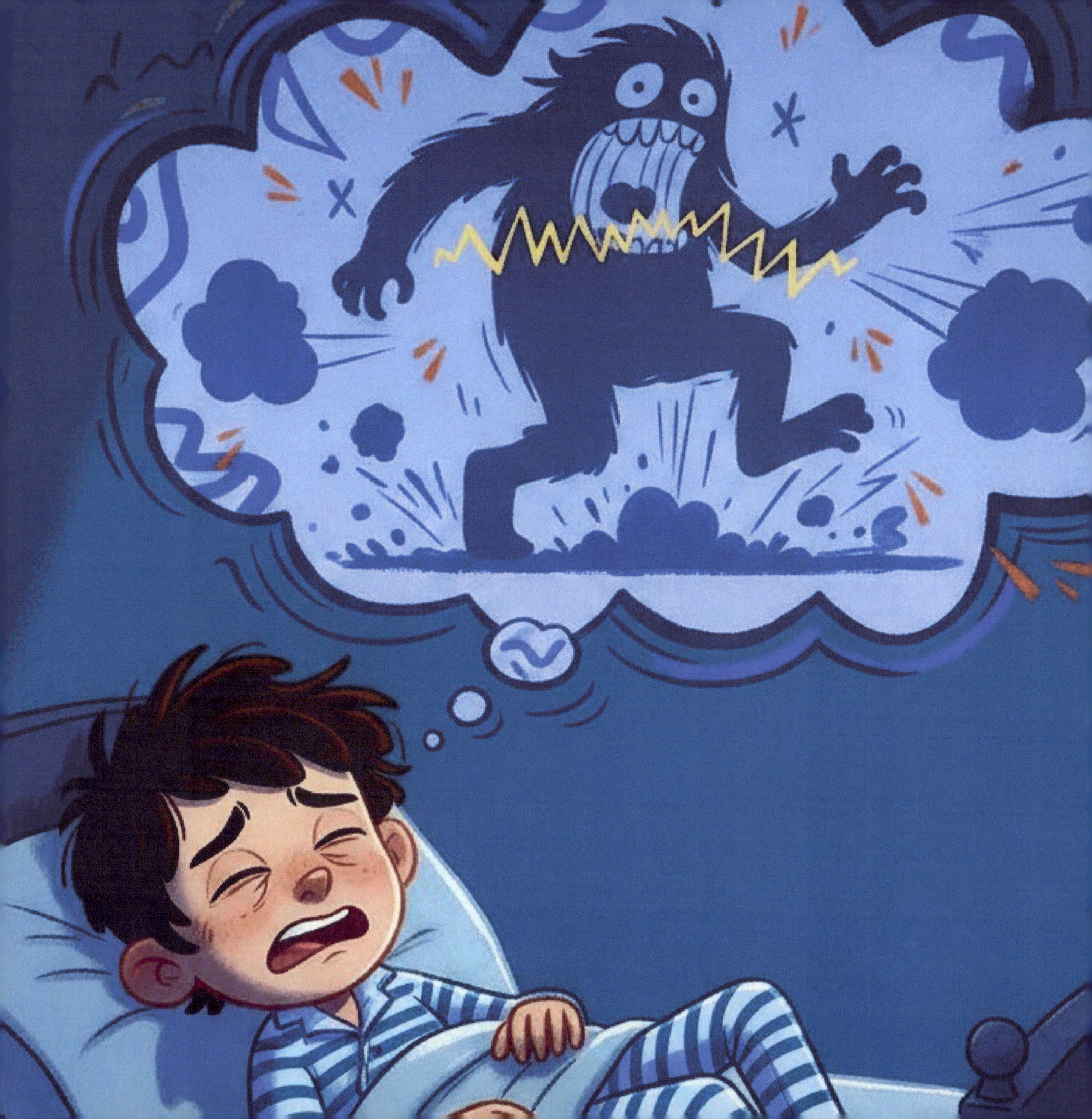

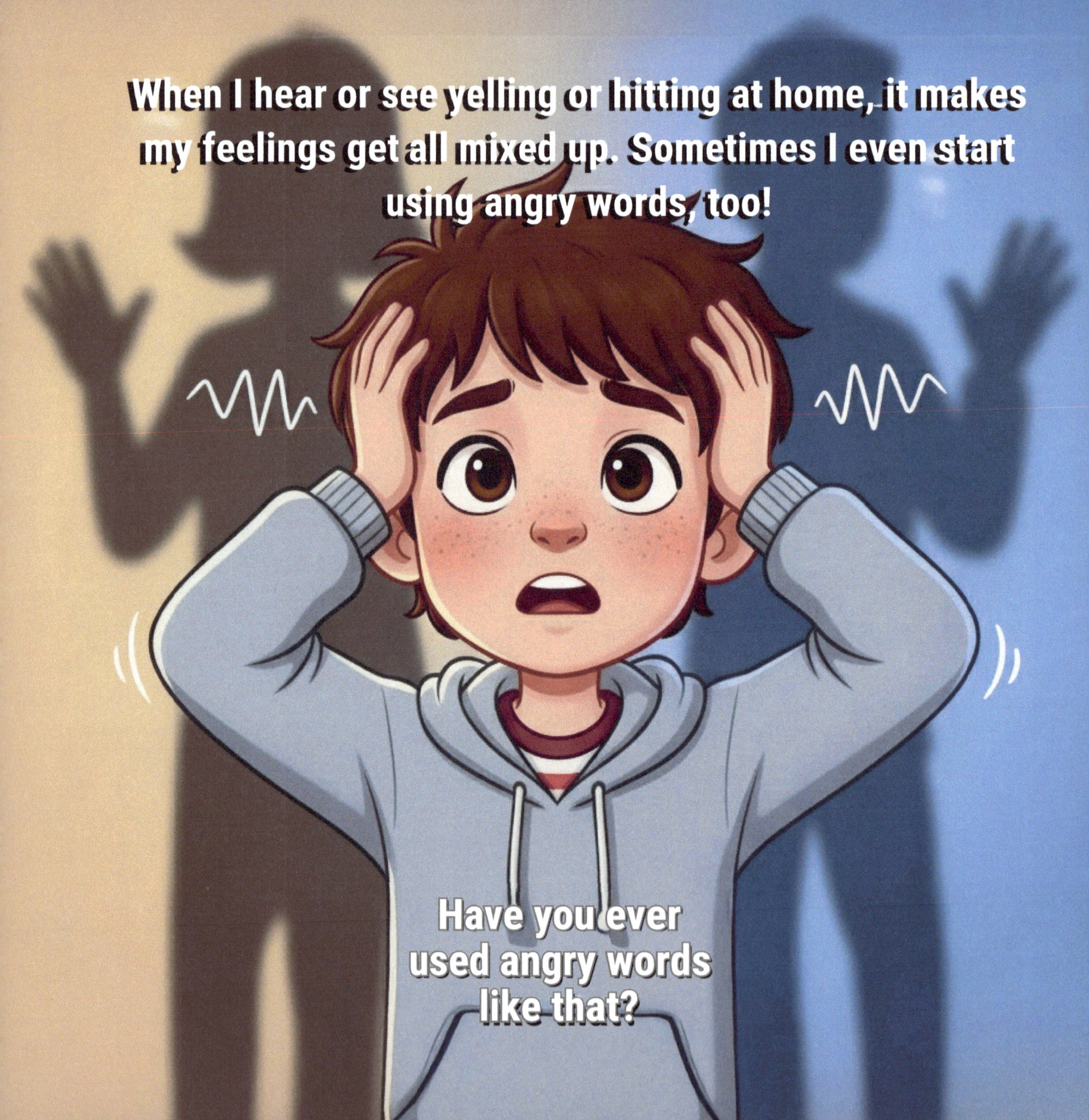

When I hear or see yelling or hitting at home, it makes my feelings get all mixed up. Sometimes I even start using angry words, too!
Have you ever used angry words like that?

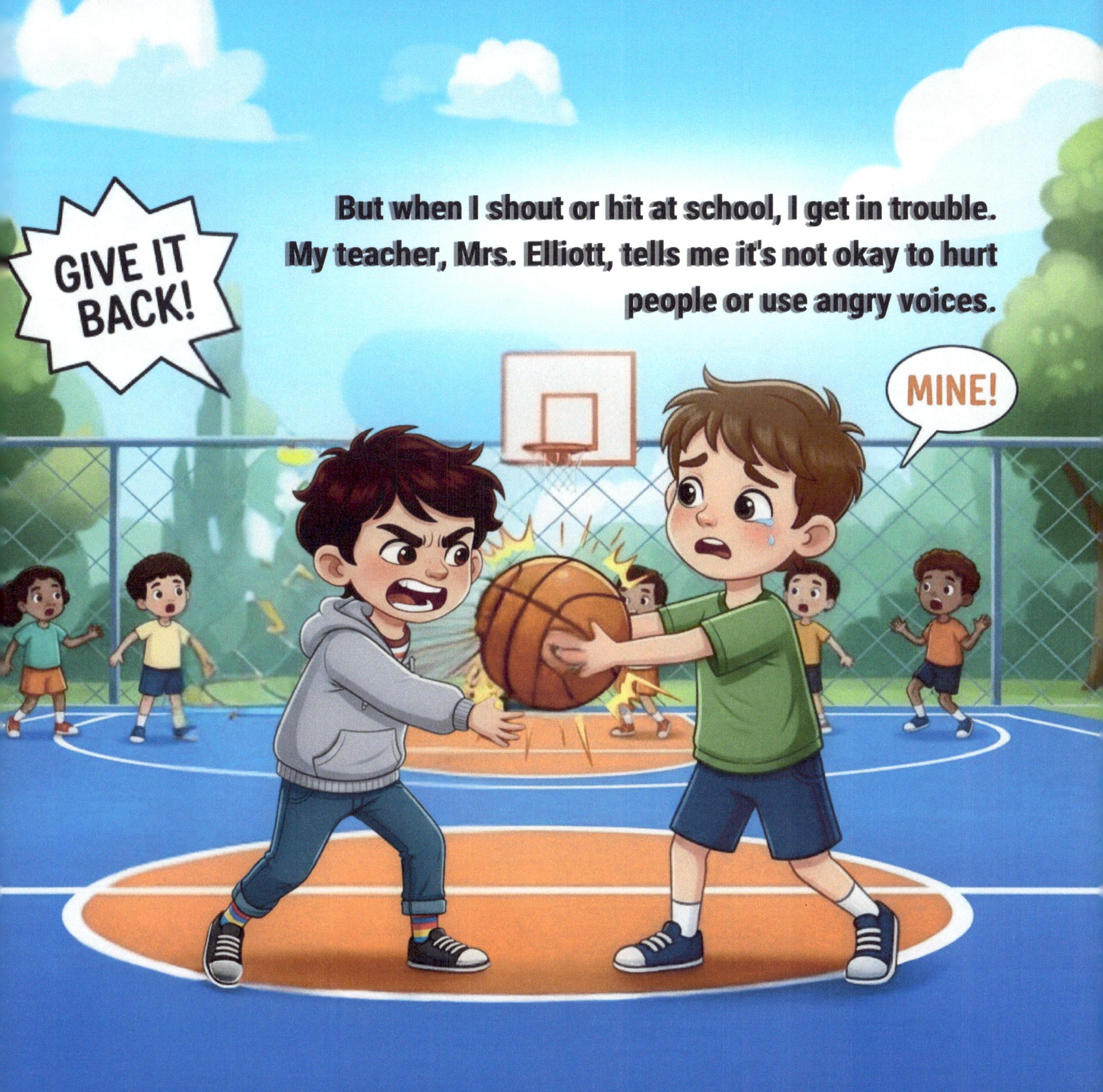

But when I shout or hit at school, I get in trouble. My teacher, Mrs. Elliott, tells me it's not okay to hurt people or use angry voices.

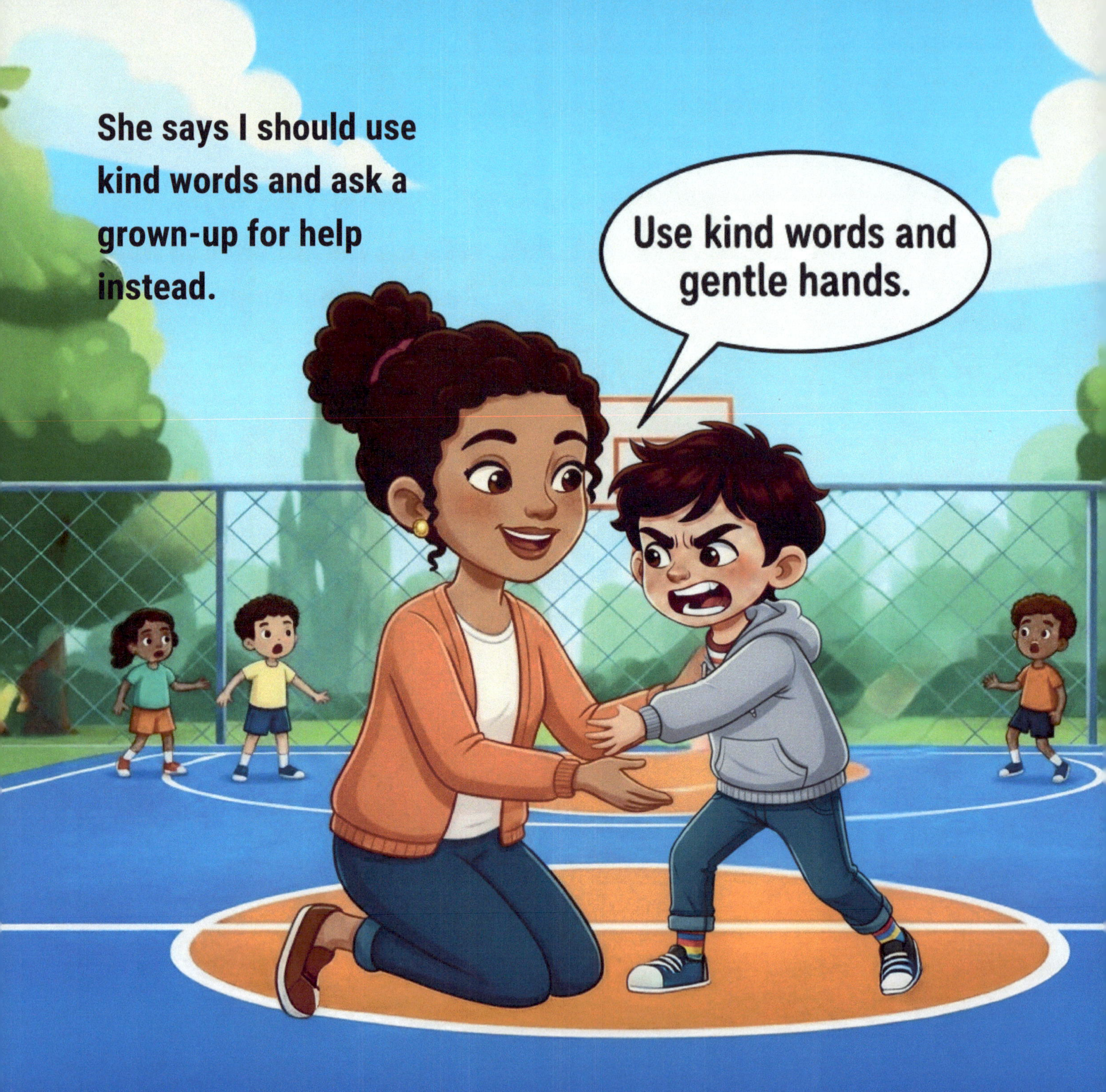
She says I should use kind words and ask a grown-up for help instead.
Use kind words and gentle hands.

Hearing yelling at home makes me feel sad. Sometimes, even when things seem okay, I don't feel like playing, eating, or laughing.

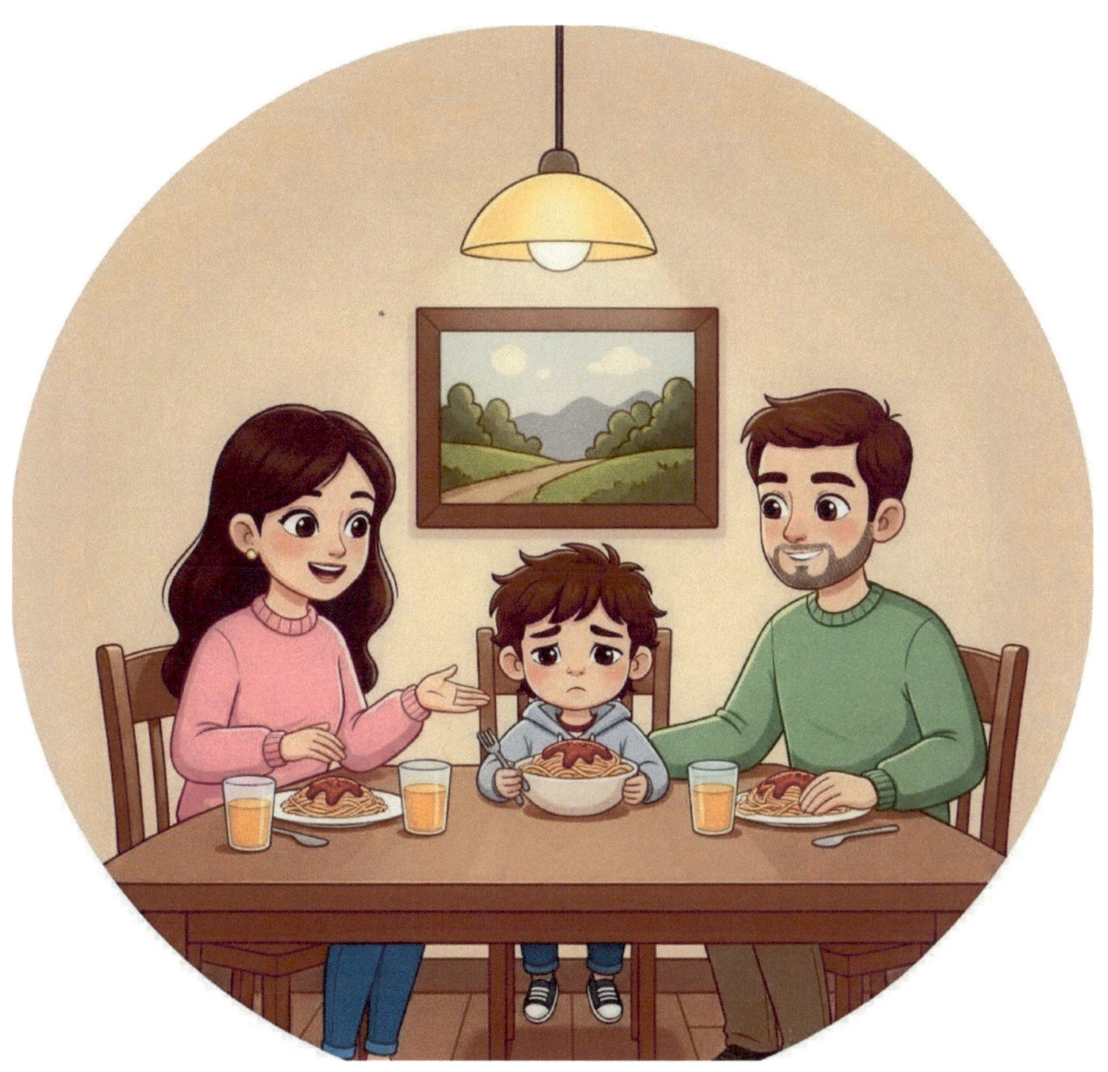

How do you think Grayson feels right now?

And sometimes, it makes me feel angry too. My face gets hot, and I imagine I'm a big dragon breathing fire everywhere!

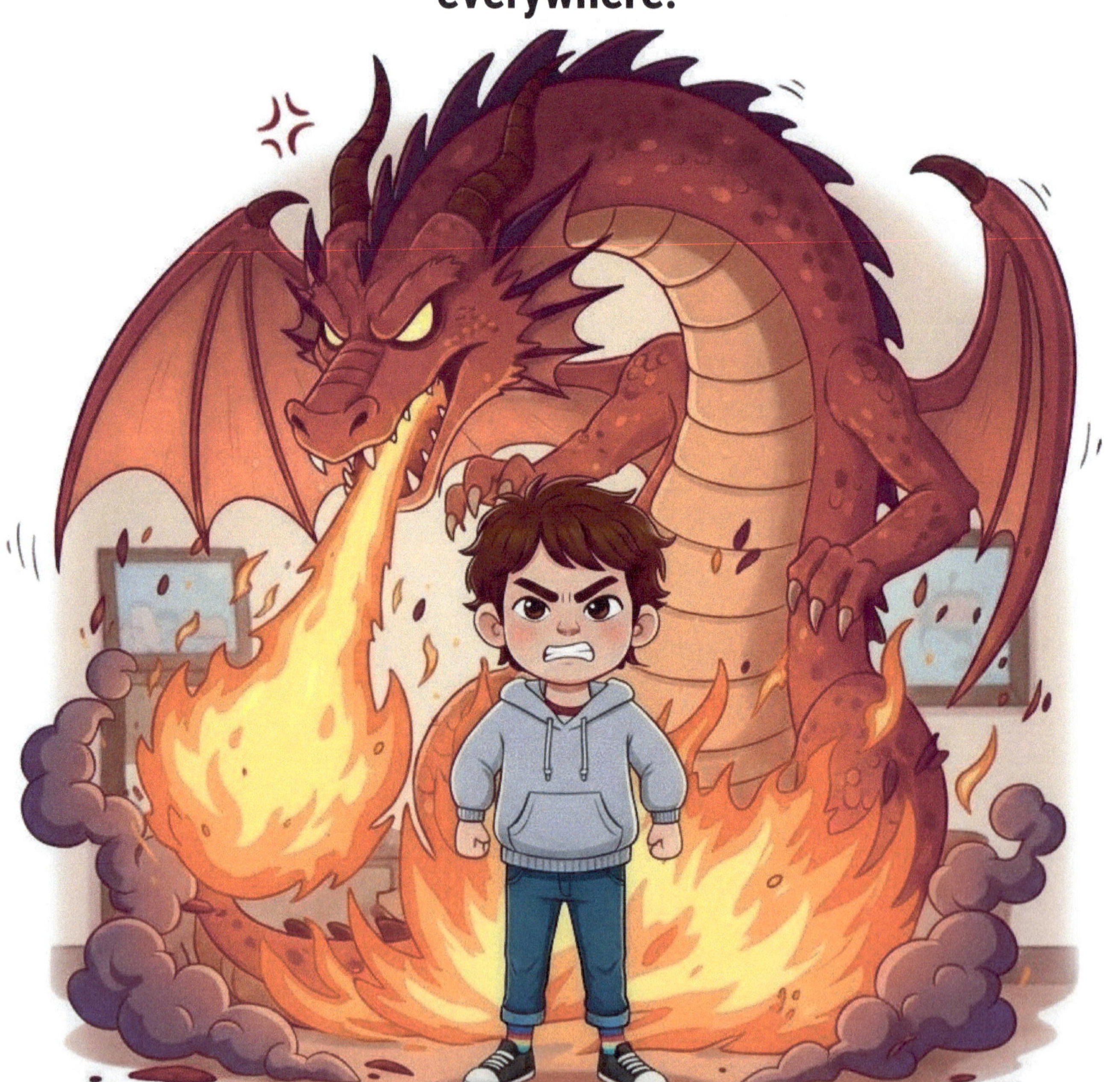

When there is yelling or hitting at home, I feel confused. I wonder if it will happen at school, too. I hope everyone will be gentle and kind.

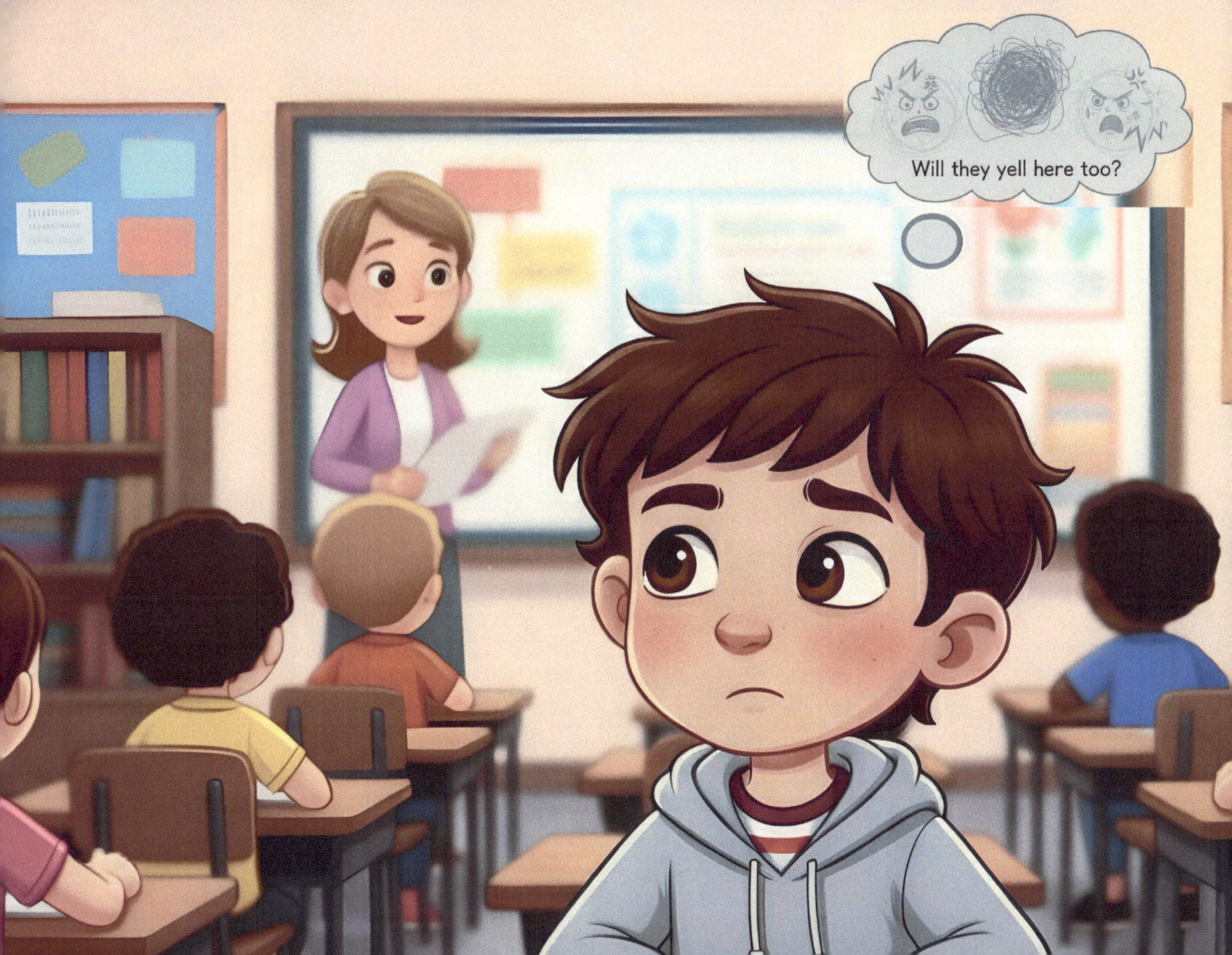

When I feel really worried, my tummy gets tight and my body feels weird. Sometimes, I even have potty accidents at school or at home.

Has that ever happend to you?

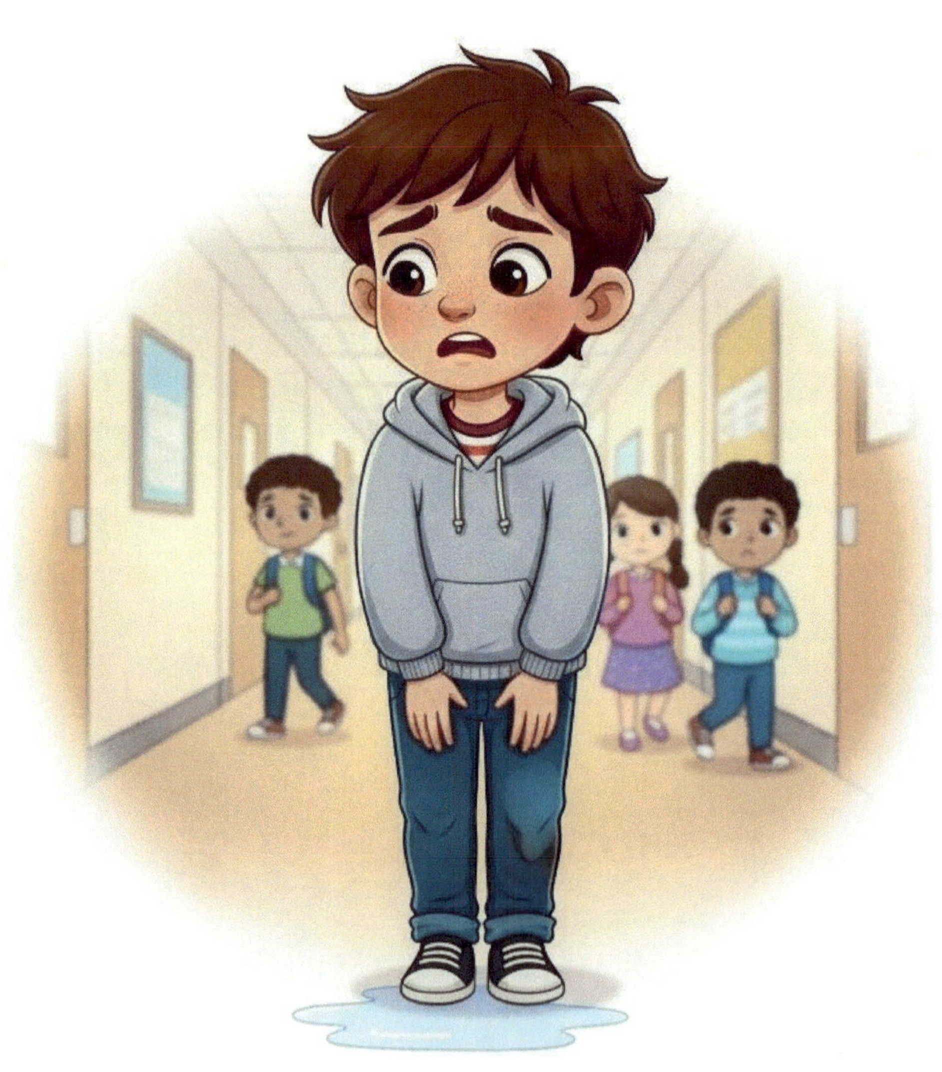

Sometimes, my mommy and daddy get upset when I have a potty accident.

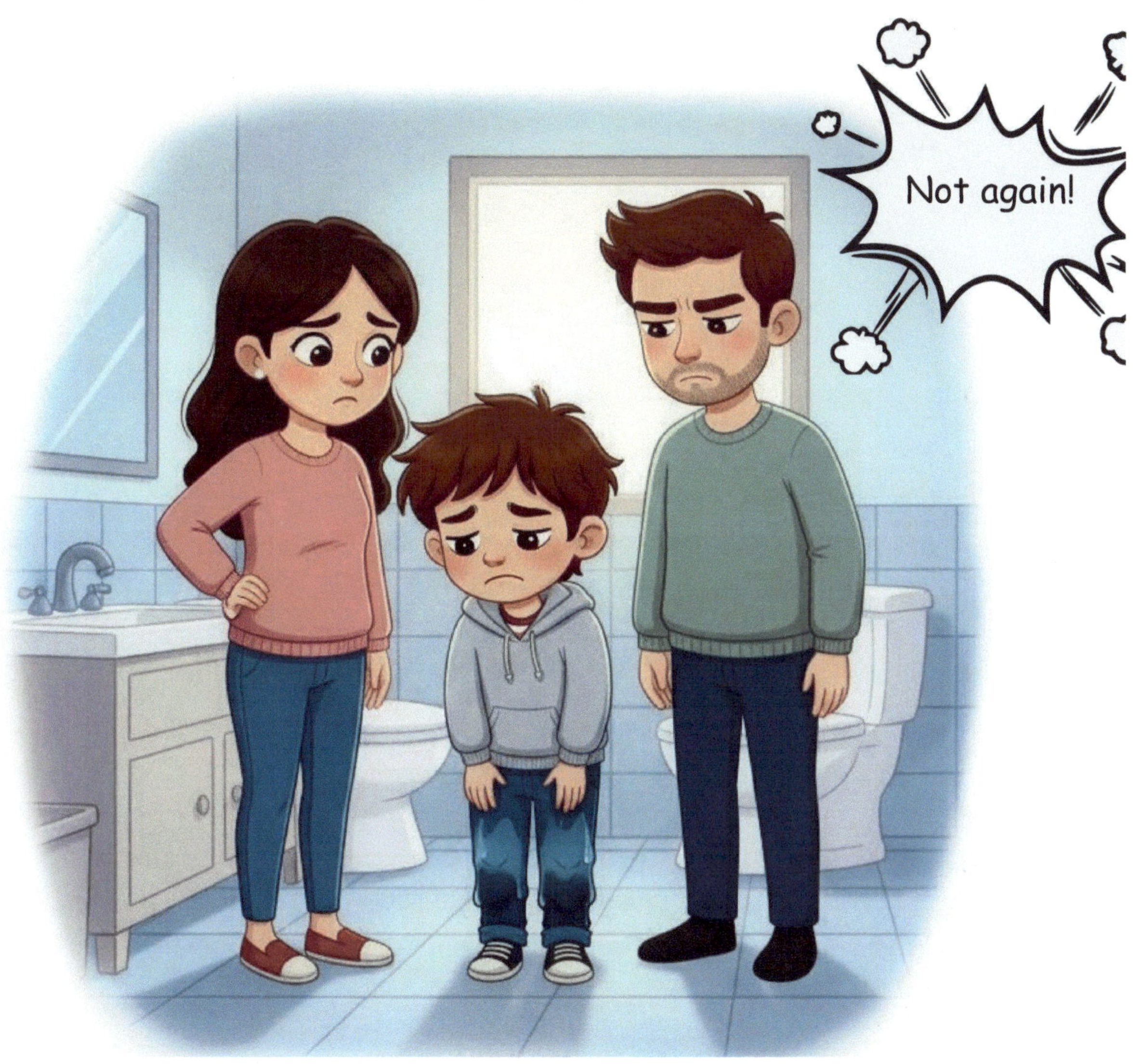

When my parents are upset with me, I feel sad.

How do you feel when your mom or dad gets mad at you?

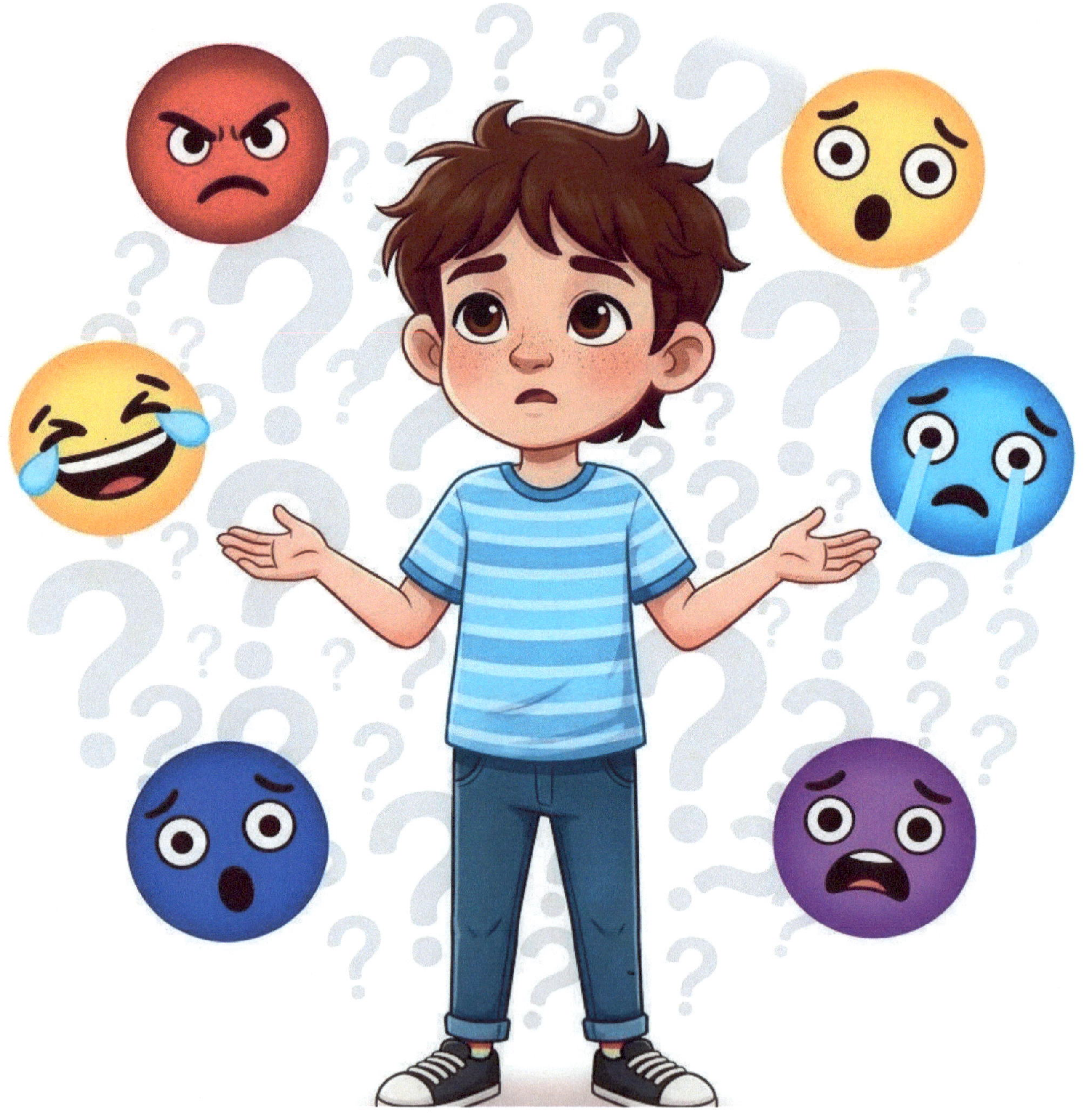

One day, I told Mommy that when people yell, it makes me feel scared and sad.

She gave me a big hug and listened to everything I was feeling.

Mommy said we needed some help,so we talked to a nice lady named Ms. Oliva. She helps families talk about feelings and teaches us how to stay safe.

Who is a grown-up you feel comfortable talking to?

Would it feel easy or hard to tell someone about your feelings?

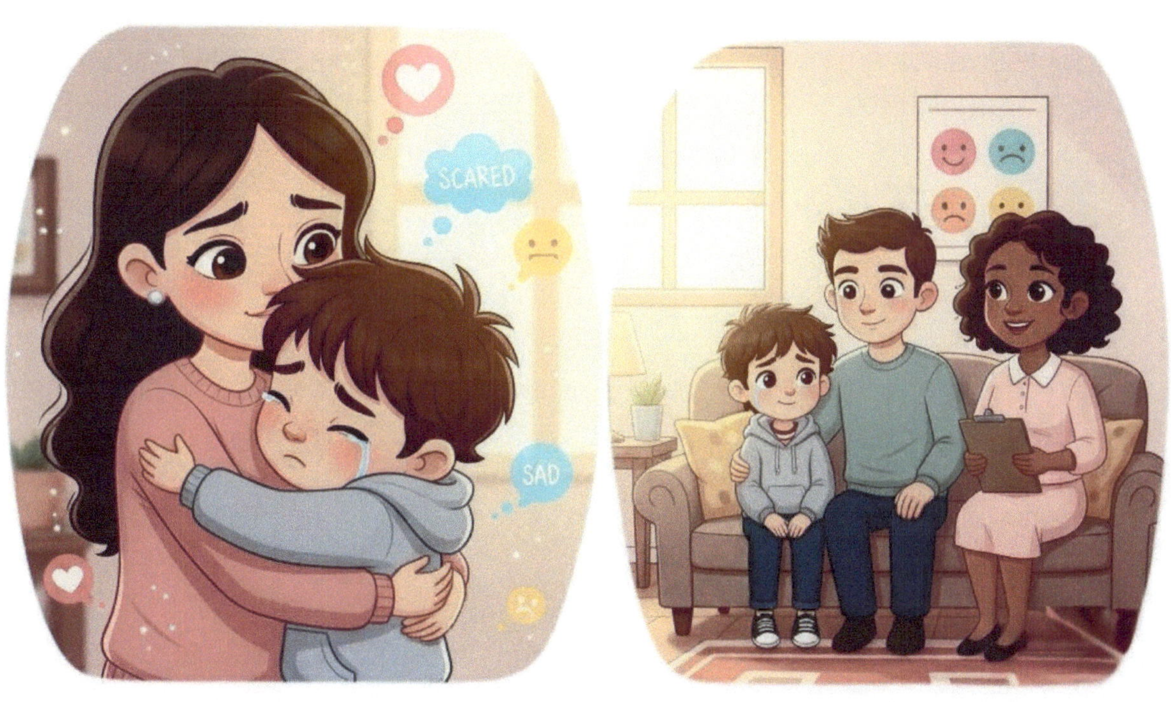

Ms. Oliva helped us make a Safety Plan.
A Safety Plan is a list of things to do to stay safe. I picked a safe room to go to when I feel scared.

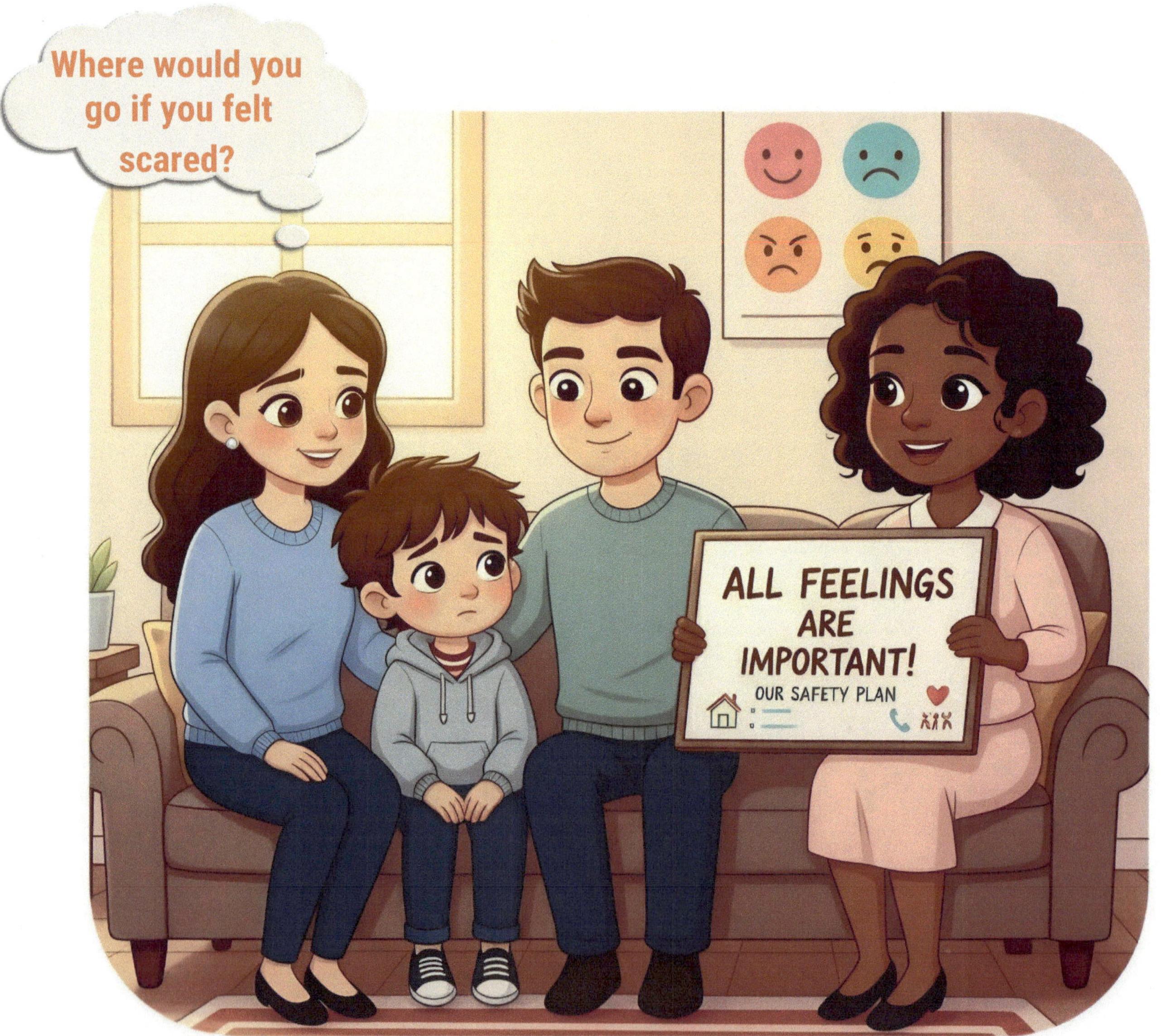

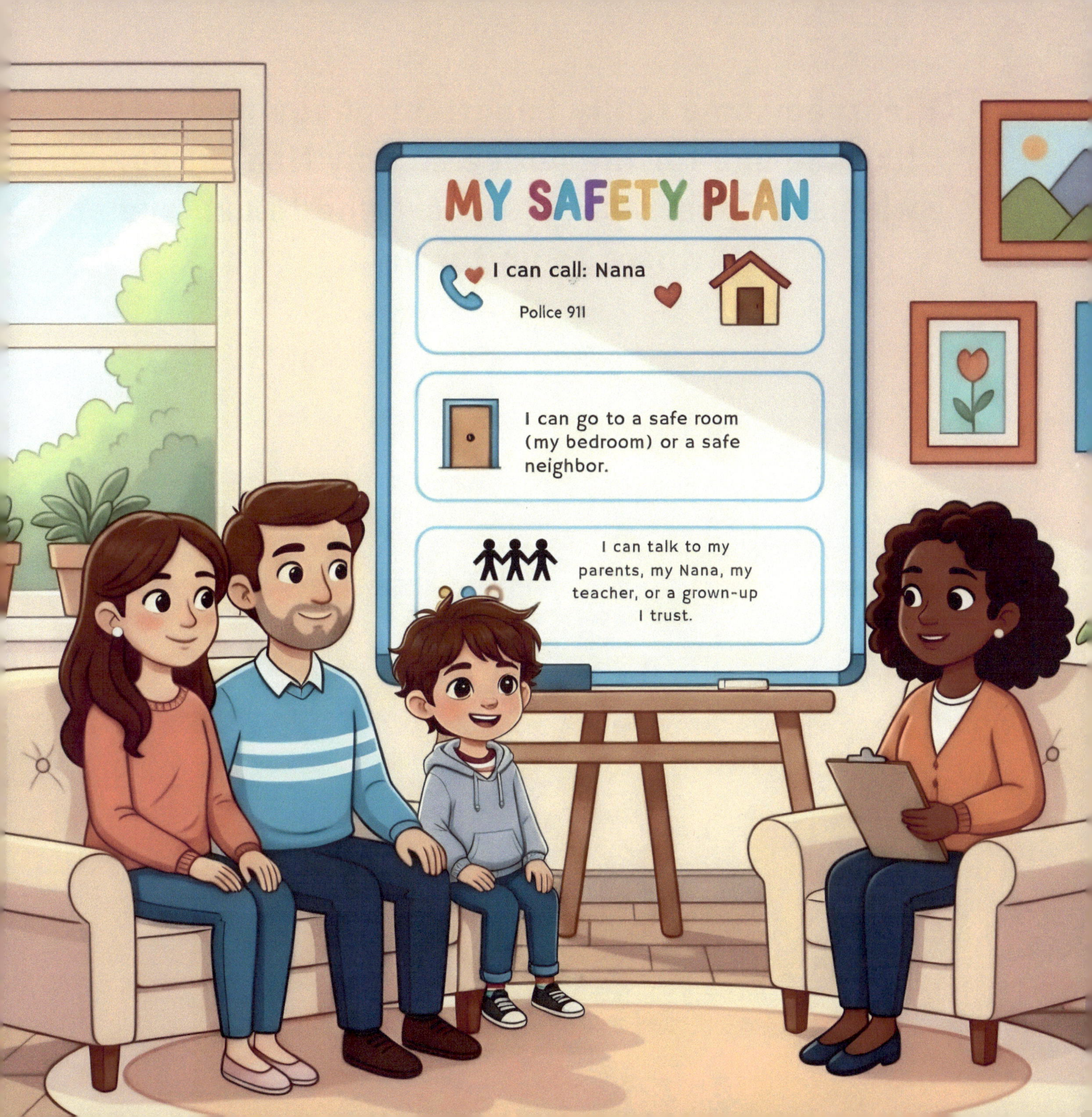

MY SAFETY PLAN
I can call: Nana
Police 911
I can go to a safe room (my bedroom) or a safe neighbor.
I can talk to my parents, my Nana, my teacher, or a grown-up I trust.

I learned some really important phone numbers, like the one for the police and my Nana's! So, whenever I get scared, I know who to call and where to go for help.

Who do you call when you're feeling scared?

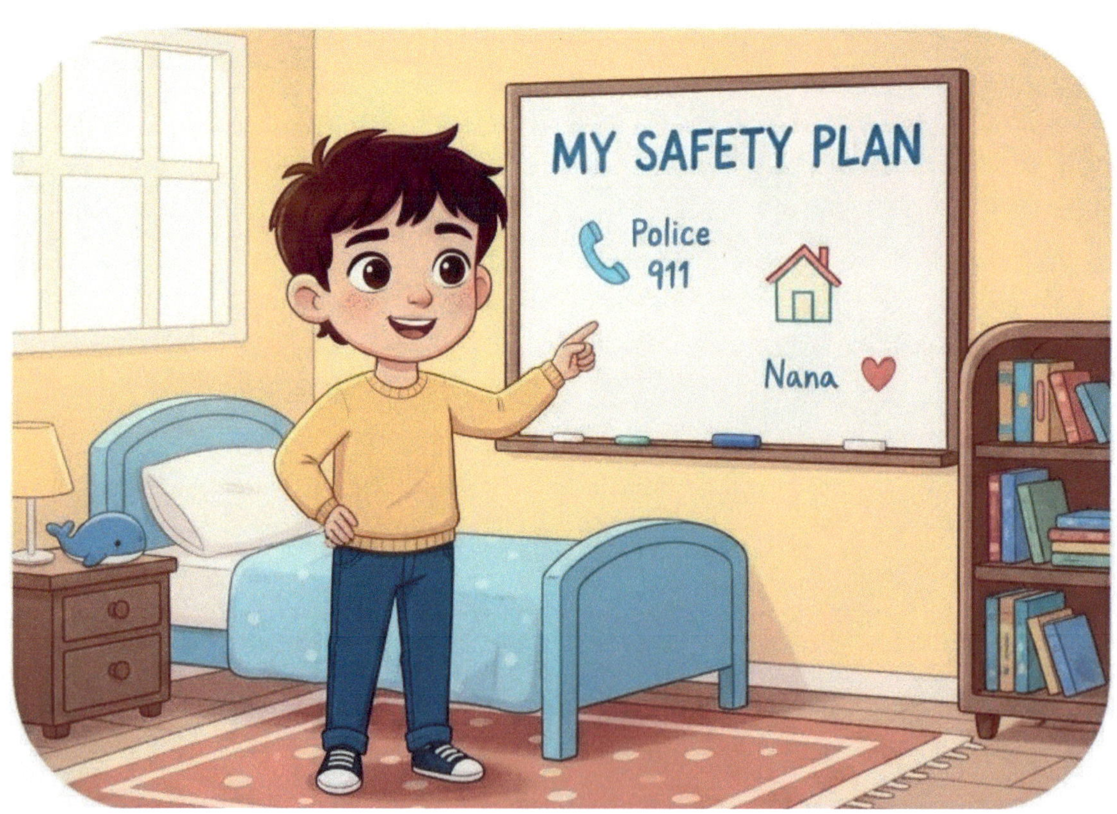

I feel safe when Mommy and Daddy help me get dry clothes and remind me it's okay to have accidents. I feel safe when they use gentle voices.

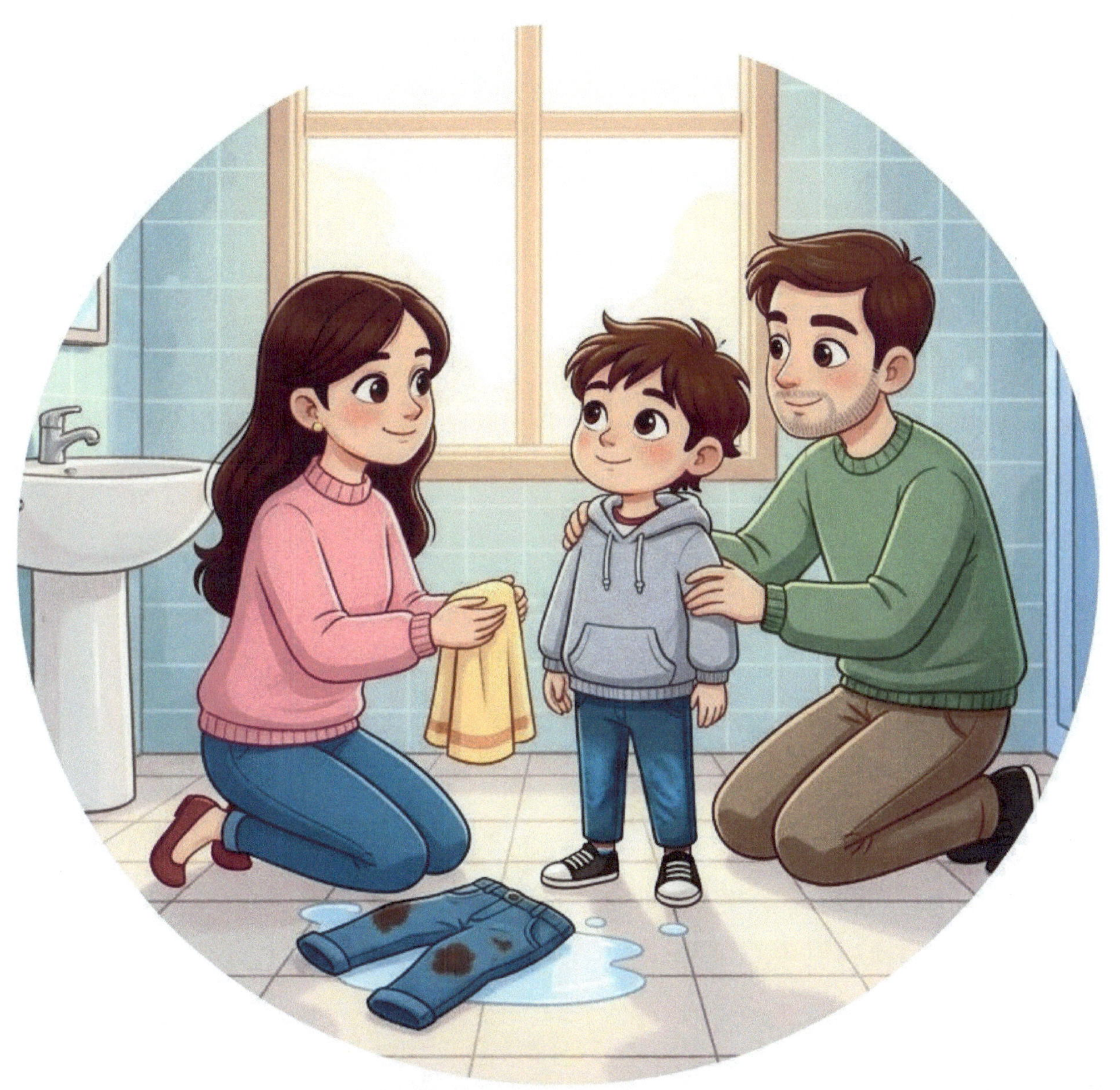

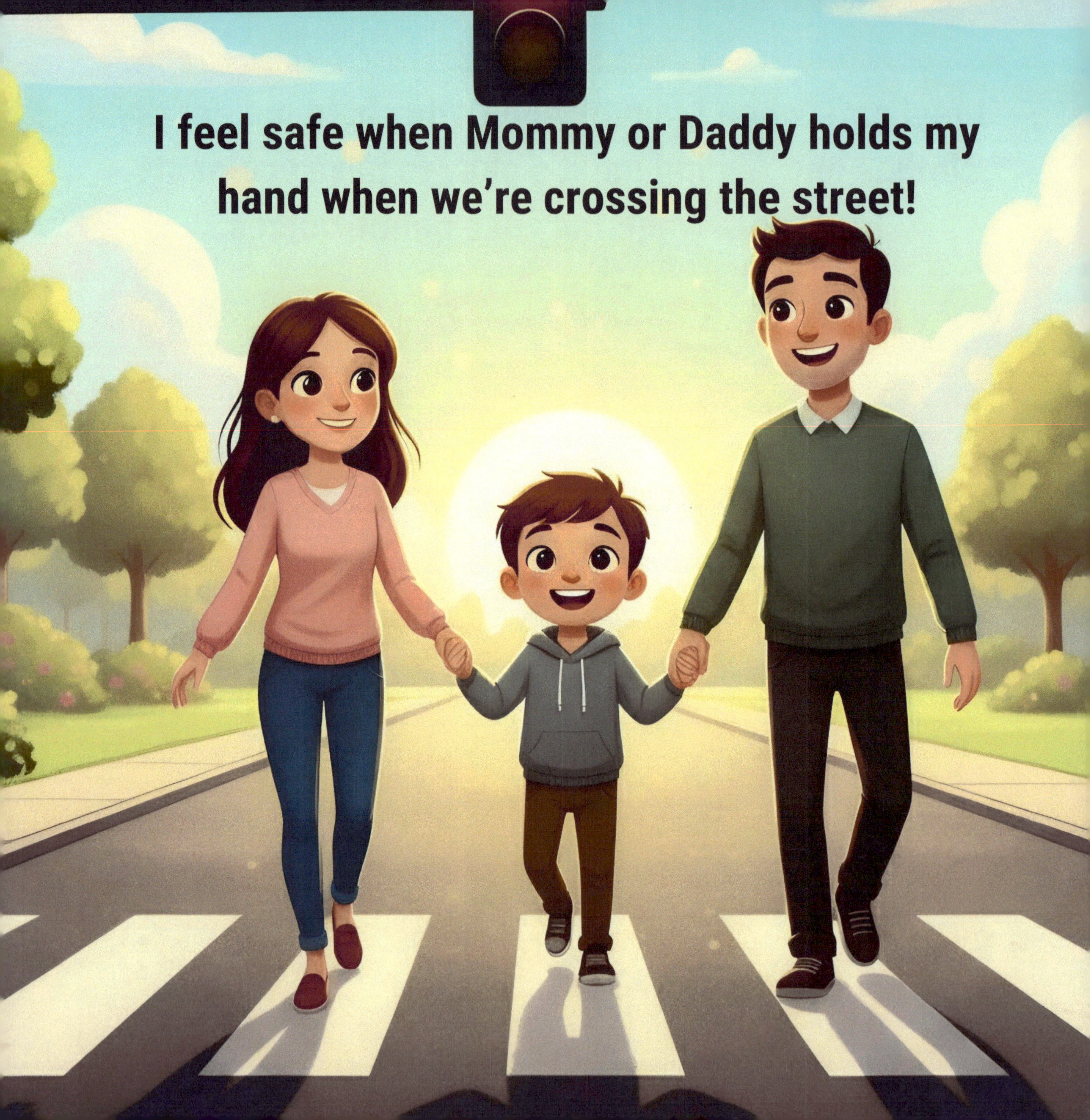

I feel safe when Mommy or Daddy holds my hand when we're crossing the street!

I feel safe when my seat belt is buckled, and driving feels smooth, not super fast.

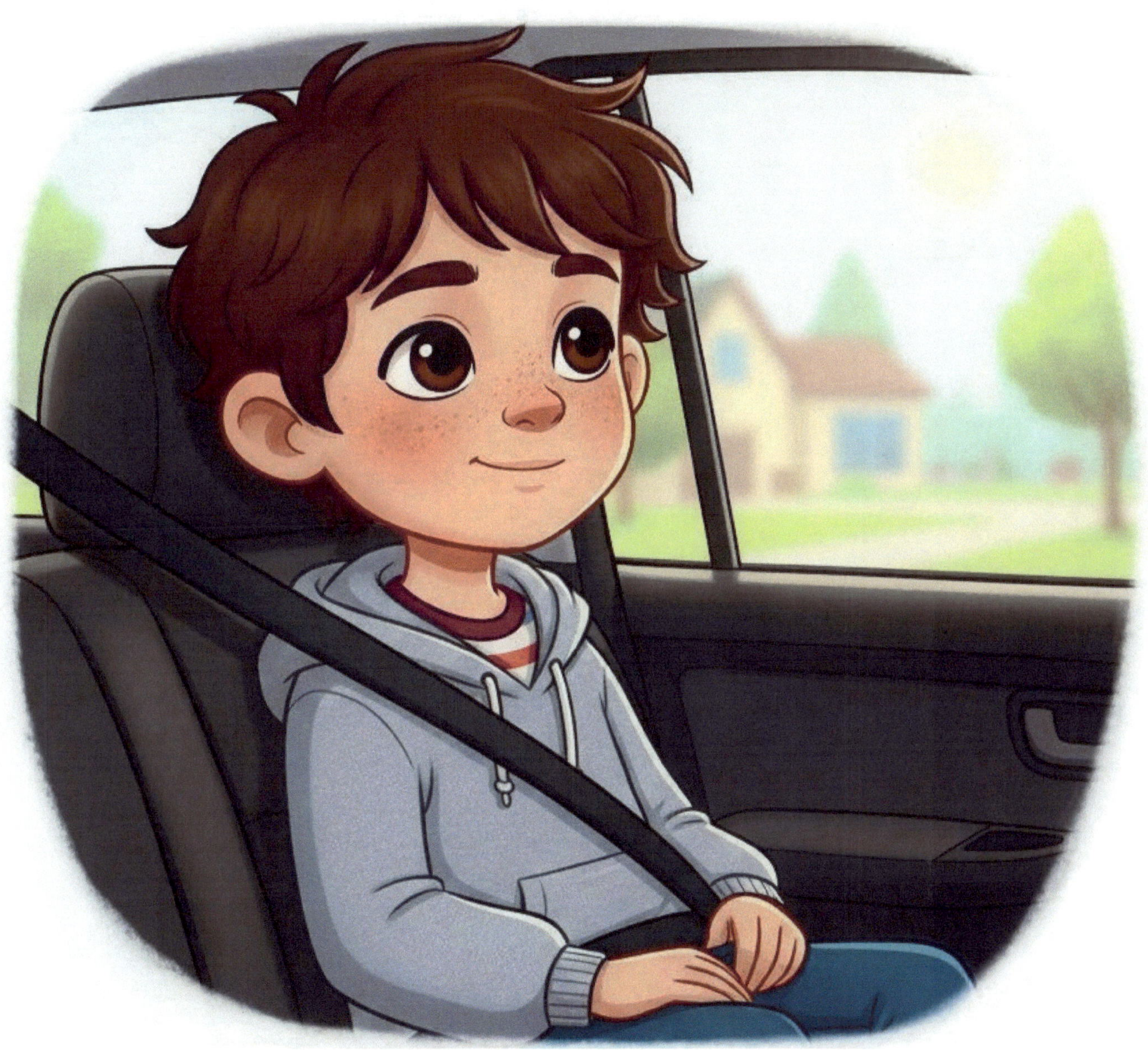

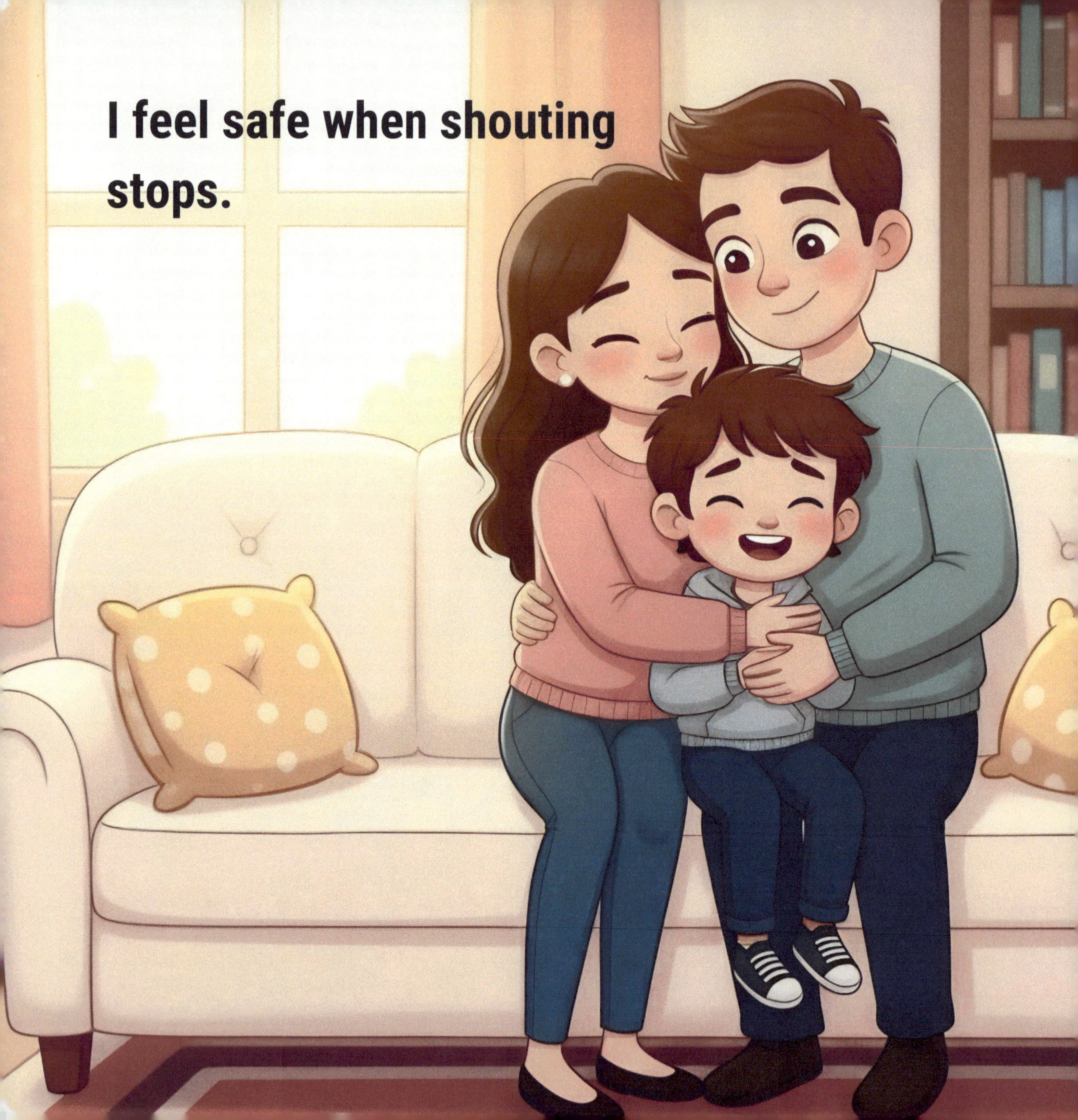
I feel safe when shouting stops.

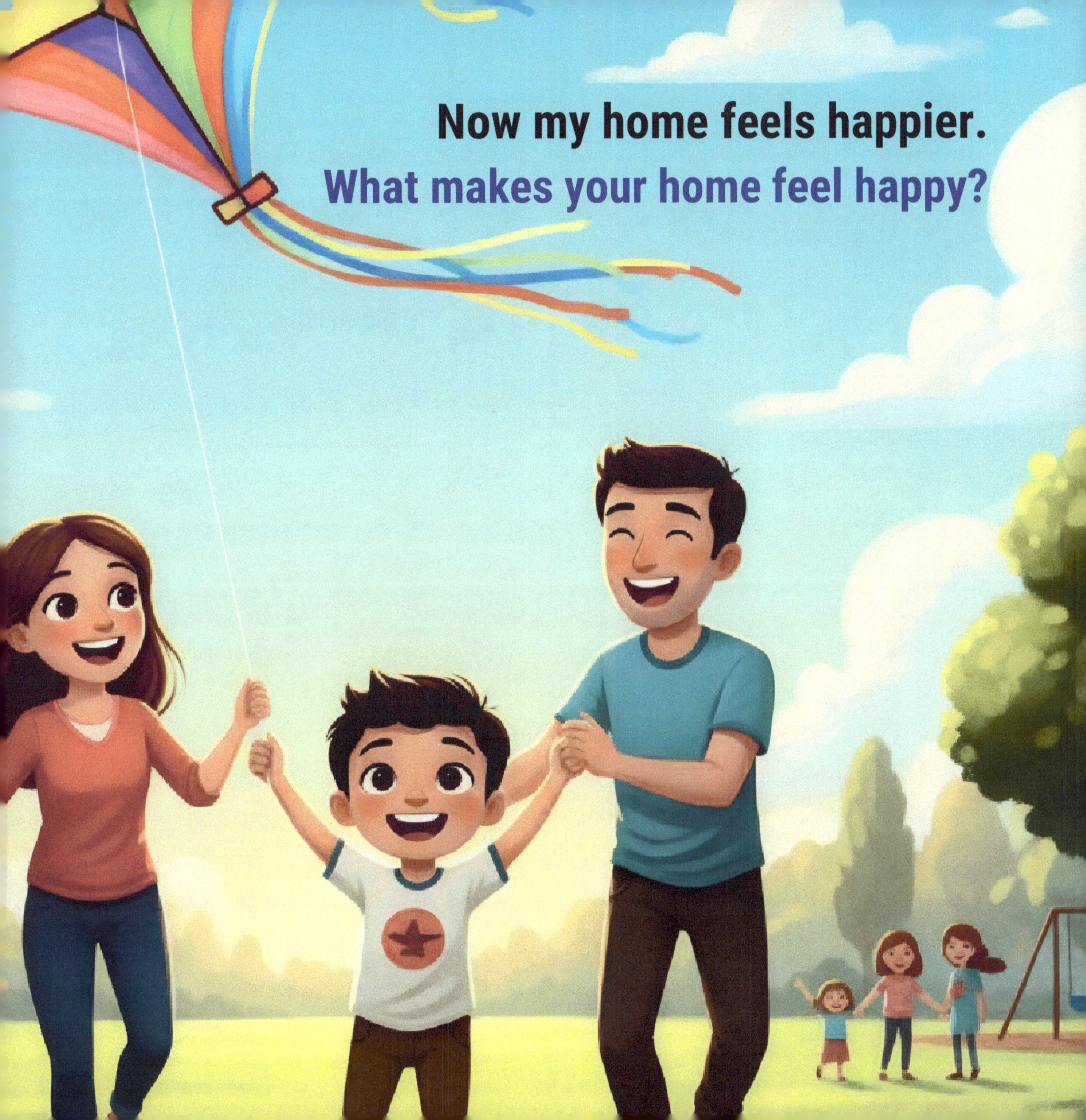

Now my home feels happier.
What makes your home feel happy?

MY SAFETY PLAN

I CAN GO TO A SAFE PLACE:

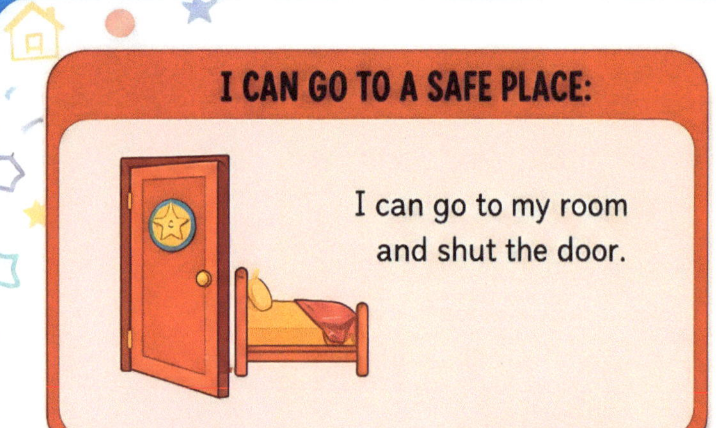

I can go to my room and shut the door.

I CAN GO SEEK HELP

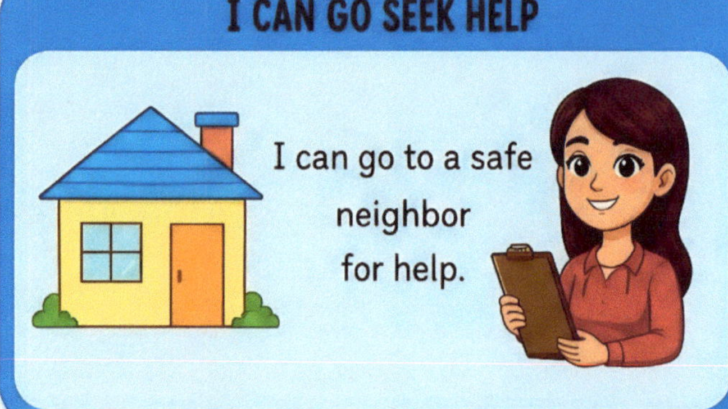

I can go to a safe neighbor for help.

I CAN GO TO A TRUSTED ADULT

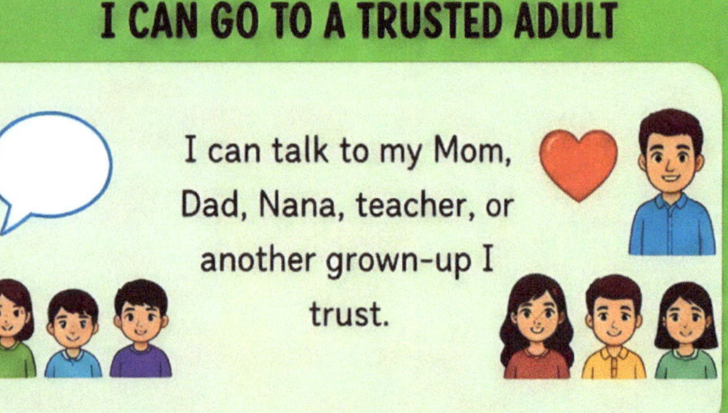

I can talk to my Mom, Dad, Nana, teacher, or another grown-up I trust.

I CAN GET HELP IMMEDIATELY

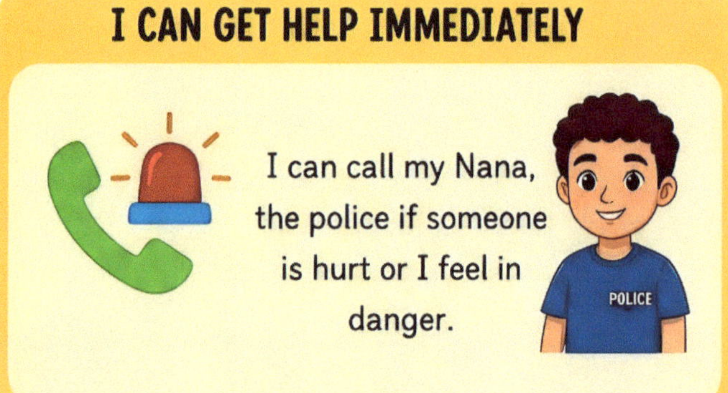

I can call my Nana, the police if someone is hurt or I feel in danger.

IMPORTANT NUMBERS TO CALL

Now I can talk about my feelings, and I know just who to go to or call when I need help:

Police/Emergency: ______________________________ USA/UK: **911 or 999**

Trusted Adult: ______________________________

Other Trusted Adult: ______________________________

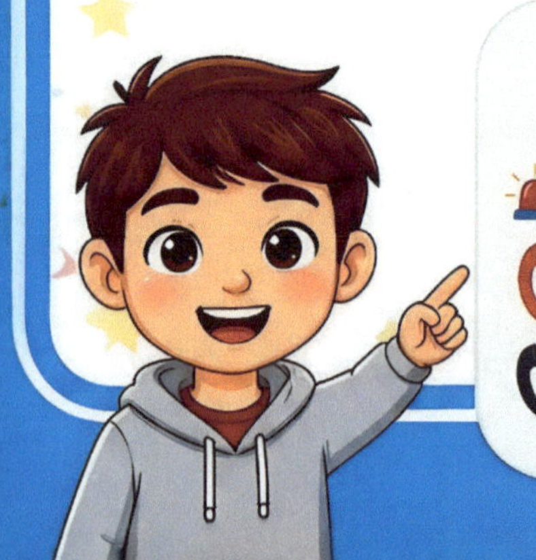

MY SAFETY PLAN

How my body feels when I'm scared:

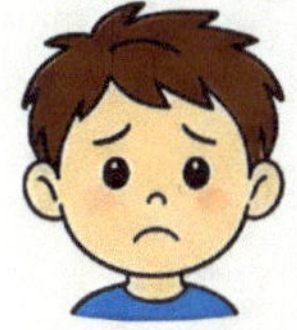 tummy tight

 fast heartbeat

 shaky

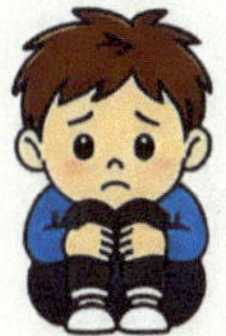 want to hide

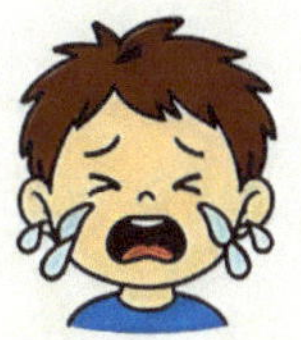 want to cry

---

What I can do when voices get loud:

- ☐ go to my safe place
- ☐ look at books or pictures
- ☐ find a safe adult
- ☐ hug my stuffed animal
- ☐ take 3 slow breaths

Important numbers I can call:

Caregiver: _______________________

Trusted adult: _______________________

Emergency: _______________________

My safety word is:

Things that make me feel safe again:

____

____

____

Now I can talk about my feelings, and I know just who to go to or call when I need help:

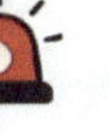 Emergency (USA): _______________________________ **Call 911**

Emergency (UK): _______________________________ **Call 999**

Trusted adult: _______________________________

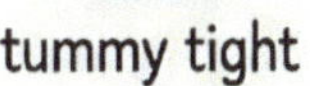

💛 Resources for Parents, Caregivers & Trusted Adults

If you or your child were impacted by this story, or if it reminded you of something happening in your home, you are not alone. Support is available—confidential, free, and without judgment.

🛑 If You or Someone Else Is in Immediate Danger

United States: Call 911 📞
United Kingdom: Call 999 📞

🏠 Domestic Violence Help & Shelter Services

United States
📞 1-800-799-SAFE (7233) | Text "START" to 88788
💻 www.thehotline.org
📞 1-800-4-A-CHILD (422-4453)
💻 www.childhelp.org

United Kingdom
📞 0808 2000 247
💻 www.nationaldahelpline.org.uk
💻 www.womensaid.org.uk
📞 0808 801 0327
💻 www.mensadviceline.org.uk

👶 Parenting & Family Support

United States
📞 1-855-427-2736
💻 www.parentsanonymous.org
📞 1-855-427-2736
💻 www.nationalparenthelpline.org
United Kingdom
📞 0808 800 2222
💻 www.familylives.org.uk
💻 www.gingerbread.org.uk

💬 Mental Health & Emotional Support

United States
📞 Text "HOME" to 741741
💻 www.crisistextline.org
www.crisistextline.org

United Kingdom
📞 Text "SHOUT" to 85258
💻 www.giveusashout.org
📞 0300 123 3393
💻 www.mind.org.uk
📞 116 123
💻 www.samaritans.org

👩🏾‍🧒🏽 Support for Children & Teens

United States
📞 1-800-422-4453
💻 www.childhelp.org

United Kingdom
📞 0800 1111
💻 www.childline.org.uk

💛 You Are Not Alone

Reading a story like this can bring up big emotions for both children and adults. Whether you're looking for advice, a safe place as to talk, or a way forward—help is out there. Healing is possible. And no matter what you've experienced, support is your right.

This list is not exhaustive—reach out locally or speak to a professional if you're unsure where to start.